Book Description

Low-Carbohydrate Intermittent Fasting (LCIF) is a natural way to live and stay healthy.

Are you tired of diet regimens that strip your body of the energy that it has by completely restricting foods that the body needs for survival and efficient functioning? You could be looking for a natural way to boost your metabolism, rejuvenate your body, and lose weight. Maybe you are searching for a way to save yourself from some bogus supplements that claim to make you look like you are half your age and embark on a more natural way to delay aging.

Would you like to follow the LCIF lifestyle but are not sure of what is involved?

Before you start intermittent fasting, you need the science-based information that explains what LCIF is. It is not one of those fad diets that are clogging the internet. Technically, LCIF is not even a diet because its focus is not on what to and what not to eat. It is focused on when to eat whatever it is that you have to eat. Learn the habit of alternate eating and fasting and let your body thank you later for it.

In *Low-Carb and Intermittent Fasting for Teens and Adults*, you will learn:

- the science behind LCIF
- how to determine whether you are overweight or not
- the benefits of LCIF
- LCIF variations and recommendations
- yummy low-carbohydrate recipes
- and so much more

It does not matter whether you have heard of intermittent fasting before or not; this book could be the door to your last stop when it comes to eating patterns. No stressful restrictions are involved. You can eat all you want and still benefit from your fasting sessions.

Like any other endeavor with benefits, LCIF is not a golden road all the way. Ups and down may occur, but these matter less when there are solutions to them. This book is your companion throughout your LCIF journey, making it as simple and fascinating as it can be.

Those that have testimonies to tell are those that dared to try. To start your journey to becoming an LCIF guru and create your own testimony, buy this book today!

Low Carb and Intermittent Fasting for Teens and Adults

A Beginner's Guide to Losing Weight, Boost Metabolism, Rejuvenate Body, and Delay Ageing the Healthy Way. Choose the Fasting Hours That Suit You.

Monica Sofia

this document is for educational and entertainment purposes only. All effort has been executed to present accurate, up to date, reliable, complete information. No warranties of any kind are declared or implied. Readers acknowledge that the author is not engaged in the rendering of legal, financial, medical or professional advice. The content within this book has been derived from various sources. Please consult a licensed professional before attempting any techniques outlined in this book.

By reading this document, the reader agrees that under no circumstances is the author responsible for any losses, direct or indirect, that are incurred as a result of the use of the information contained within this document, including, but not limited to, errors, omissions, or inaccuracies.

Table of Contents

Introduction

The internet is clogged with various ways to lose weight and maintain one's desired weight, but do they all work? The answer is a resounding "No." Usually, people turn to different diet and exercise regimens, some of which seem to work during the early days of practicing them. The truth of the matter is that most of the time, they do not work in the long run.

As technological advances continue to rise, lifestyles progressively become oriented to the sedentary. People have more screen time, to the extent that time to sleep is drastically reduced, as they don't sleep till toward or after the heart of the night. A lot of online jobs have emerged, and people are increasingly working from home. The better part of the day is spent sitting down, in front of a desktop or laptop. Communication has shifted from more physical interaction to online social platforms. Everything is just a click away, even food, as online ordering platforms are becoming more and more popular. The route to the bank has been replaced by a few clicks on your smartphone or tablet.

Such inactive lifestyles, coupled with unmonitored eating habits, are a quick way to bring additional calories onboard. When these calories are not burned in one way or another, one may become overweight, and the risk of diseases such as type 2 diabetes is quite elevated. Inadequate sleep is also another ingredient to being obese. When you follow poor sleeping patterns, you have less leptin—the hormone that informs you to stop eating more food (Mann, 2013). In most cases, when leptin levels decrease, the level of ghrelin, the hunger hormone, increases, leading to the urge to eat more. To add on to that, limited sleep reduces the rate of metabolism. Less of the food that you eat will be metabolized when your metabolism occurs at a slower rate, and this causes obesity.

Even with limited exercise, probably due to busy schedules that are characteristic of the 21st century, you can still monitor your weight, eat healthily, and shield yourself from diseases that result from eating disorders. A low-carbohydrate diet coupled with intermittent fasting will do the trick and leave you more energetic and focused, without the fatigue that results from fat accumulation.

Intermittent fasting is a unique approach to healthy eating. Most diets focus on what to and what not to eat, which is usually difficult to stick to, especially when the recommended diet requires that one trims off some of the food that was part of their previous diets. It takes time to make the new diet part of one's lifestyle. On the contrary, intermittent fasting pivots on when to eat your food, not necessarily what you should eat. As a result, one might not need to change their dietary patterns, but there is ample time for the food to be metabolized and used up during the fasting hours.

In this book, we are going to couple intermittent fasting and a lower carbohydrate diet to ensure that you stay healthy. You will be furnished with information that is supported by scientific evidence to confirm its efficacy. Not only will you learn how to stick to the low carbohydrate diet and intermittent fasting, but you will also get a bonus of 10 yummy recipes that you can try as you embark on this worthwhile journey. Enjoy!

Chapter 1: Low Carb and Intermittent Fasting (LCIF) Defined

Intermittent fasting involves a regular schedule which alternates between eating and fasting. Fasting simply means intentionally refraining from food until the scheduled time for eating. On the other hand, a low-carbohydrate diet is self-explanatory. A low-carbohydrate diet restricts the inclusion and consumption of foods that are rich in carbohydrates, primarily starchy and sugary foods. Instead of eating carbohydrate-dominant foods like bread and pasta, one can use whole foods to replace them. This chapter is dedicated to dissecting the concepts surrounding LCIF.

Intermittent Fasting

As highlighted earlier on, intermittent fasting does not pinpoint the foods that you should eat, but rather when you should eat whatever you choose to eat. Intermittent fasting is, therefore, less of a diet and more of an eating pattern.

Although it has only recently gained popularity, intermittent fasting is an ancient practice. Since time immemorial, the hunter-gatherers would go through unplanned intermittent fasting because food was not always available. Even in current generations, people who subscribe to the Christian and Islamic religions, for example, do fast. The only difference with the previously mentioned fasting method is that it is for spiritual reasons. The intermittent fasting that we are focusing on in this book is for health reasons.

The Science Behind Intermittent Fasting

Normally, your body depends on the food that you eat during your meals for it to carry out all the bodily functions that enhance survival. All body processes require energy that is produced by the body through respiration, which also needs glucose to take place. In fact, the survival of every cell that makes up your body is accredited to the process of respiration.

When you eat your food, it goes through digestion, where it is broken down into smaller-sized molecules, a process which increases the surface area of the food molecules. Remember, the smaller the molecules, the larger the surface area and vice versa. The larger surface area on the food molecules enhances more efficient absorption of food components, such as carbohydrates, fats, proteins, and vitamins, into the bloodstream. From there, the food components are distributed throughout the body for their respective functions.

It is, however, important to note that blood glucose levels are highly controlled. There are certain amounts of glucose that the blood can contain at any given time, even though these levels are usually exceeded soon after eating. How then does the body reduce the levels of glucose to permissible ones? The pancreas secretes a hormone called insulin that regulates the concentrations of glucose that should be available in the body at any given time. In the event that the glucose levels in the blood are too high, insulin triggers the processes that convert the "extra" glucose to glycogen. Glycogen molecules are made up of glucose molecules, logically merged together, and they are stored in the liver and the muscles.

The glycogen in the liver can be broken down to glucose and released into the bloodstream if blood glucose levels subside below the normal levels. This process is regulated by glucagon, a hormone that is produced by the pancreas. The glycogen stored in the muscles is only used by the muscle cells, especially during activity.

The liver and muscles keep limited amounts of glycogen, which is usually for short-term needs. If there is still extra glucose after these glycogen stores are created, it is converted to fat, which you can picture as the long-term storage form of glucose (Fletcher, 2010). This storage is your last resort source of energy that enables you to pull through many days without eating. Now, when you eat your meals regularly, there is a greater probability that you will pile up the fat reserves because the bloodstream is rarely in need of glucose from the liver and sometimes the muscles. Therefore, most of your glucose will be stored as fat, and this continuous cycle will lead to obesity.

When you undergo intermittent fasting, you give your body the time to use up the glucose that you ate in your last meal. Depending on how long your fasting will be and how much glycogen you have stored up, the glycogen stores in the liver may be depleted so that your body reaches out to the fat stores for energy. The glucose for energy is released through the breakdown of fats, a process called adipolysis. That way, your next meal will not simply heap up fat stores but first attend to the blood glucose requirements, as well as liver and muscle glycogen stores. Therefore, intermittent fasting is a great way to monitor fat accumulation in your body and prevent the diseases that are linked to obesity, such as type 2 diabetes. It does this by prolonging the time required to burn any extra calories so that you keep healthy.

A Low-Carb Diet Hastens Weight Loss. Why?

The research niche that explores the impacts of several diet regimens on weight loss is increasingly gaining attention. Evidence that supports the efficacy of the low-carb diet in aiding weight loss is also accumulating. In one study, the researchers compared the effects of a low-fat, low-carb, and Mediterranean diet on weight loss and maintenance (Shai et al., 2008). After two years' results, analysis showed that the low-carb diet and Mediterranean diets were efficacious in reducing and maintaining weight.

Low Calorie In, High Calorie Out

Calories refer to the energy in food, and it is usually presented to the body in the form of glucose. When the number of calories that you eat surpasses the energy requirements of the body, all extra calories are stored as fat. This increases your body weight.

The more calories you consume through your food, the greater the chances of gaining weight. By simply reducing the amount of carbohydrates that you consume, you cut down on the calories that you take into your body. There are average amounts of calories that the body uses up each day, and that amount is what is referred to as "calorie out." You can even increase the "calorie out" amounts by engaging in activities that require a lot of energy, such as exercising. The idea that is presented in this section is that you should consume fewer calories than the ones that you will burn out. That way, you reduce weight. Burning an average of 750 calories per day from your diet yields a loss of approximately one pound (0.5 kilograms) within a week (Mayo Clinic Staff, 2020).

Manipulating the Thermic Effect of Food (TEF)

Low-carbohydrate diets do not focus on the protein sources, but rather the carbohydrate sources. This implies that while you reduce the amount of carbohydrates that you take in, your protein intake may remain less monitored. Having explained that, it is of paramount importance that you understand that the energy that is required to burn calories from different food components is never the same. This means that more work and energy is required to digest, absorb, metabolize and assimilate some foods, than is needed for others (Petre, 2019). The amount of work and energy that is required to completely metabolize a certain type of food is quantified in terms of the thermic effect of food (TEF).

Foods that requisite more energy for them to be fully metabolized have a high TEF. Proteins have a high TEF, as compared to fats and carbohydrates. More calories are used up in the process of metabolizing proteins, than those that are burned when processing other food components. So, when you eat a low-carb diet and eat more protein, you increase the number of calories that are needed to burn the food, as many of the calories will be used to burn the protein. You will have reduced the calorie intake by eating fewer carbohydrates, which are the main source of calories, while you burn more of these calories to process the protein. Doing the math will leave you realizing that the low-carb diet greatly reduces available calories in the body. The end result is weight loss because of the reduced availability of calories that aid weight gain.

Slowing Down the Processing

Diets that are high in carbohydrates, especially those with lower fiber like white rice and white bread, are processed at a faster rate. They do not stay longer in the digestive system because of their simple nature. However, when the amounts of these carbohydrates are lowered and coupled with, say, proteins, the processing rate is far slower, keeping you fuller for longer (Vanderwall, n.d.). The implication of this is that you are less likely to get hungry more frequently, so you reduce the possibility of eating more calories through abnormally frequent meals.

Reducing the Glucose-to-Fat Conversion

A high-carb diet causes surges in blood sugar levels, which triggers the secretion of more insulin. While the intention of insulin is to maintain blood sugar levels within normal ranges, its actions lead to the conversion of some of the glucose to fat, which is a weight gain factor. In people who are hyperglycemic, weight gain may result from insulin resistance. Hyperglycemia is a condition where one has prolonged high blood glucose levels. When cells of the body become unresponsive to insulin, this is called insulin resistance, and it leads to a rise in sugar and insulin levels. Despite the fact that the cells don't respond to insulin in terms of taking up glucose, they respond to it in terms of storing the glucose as fat (Kubala, 2019). This also causes weight gain. However, when added sugars are reduced in alignment with a low-carb diet, issues such as insulin resistance are less expected, ultimately avoiding weight gain. Sometimes, the best way to lose weight is by reducing weight gain.

Myths and Facts About Intermittent Fasting

Some people resent fasting for many reasons. Some simply can't imagine themselves not eating when food is available, while some act in response to the myths that they have heard concerning the practice. It is important to note that myths are not facts and can be misleading. In this section, you will be able to demarcate between the myths and facts of intermittent fasting.

1. **Myth:** All types of intermittent fasting have the same results as continuous dieting procedures, only that the former is far less comfortable.

   Facts: First, not everyone struggles with fasting; some do not. Besides, just like some strict diets, fasting may take some time to learn and master. Your body will become increasingly comfortable with the fasting procedure with time. Second, there is no "one size fits all" rule for intermittent fasting. The fasting hours differ with each type. While one may not be comfortable with one method of intermittent fasting, they may find another one that is more relevant to their lifestyle and schedules.

2. **Myth:** Fasting causes binging and overeating because you will be hungry after your fast.

Facts: Binging and overindulging are eating disorders that are not tied to fasting. Self-control is what one needs in order to stop overindulging, not refraining from fasting. In most cases, people who fast more tend to eat less in the long run.

3. **Myth:** Intermittent fasting is for all people.

   Facts: Intermittent fasting is a beneficial practice, but that does not make it suitable for everyone. It is not recommended for pregnant women, children, underweight people, and those with specific underlying chronic conditions that require that they eat before they take their medications. Children cannot fast because they are in periods of rapid growth and so they need adequate nutrients to cater for the growth needs. The same applies to pregnant women; their unborn children need all the nutrients for optimal growth.

4. **Myth:** Fasting lowers your metabolic rate at rest. Since the number of calories that your body will burn while you are at rest is reduced, you will gain more weight once you start eating normally again.

   Facts: Some diets, especially those that limit calorie intake, impact the rate of metabolism, reducing it to suit the lower energy intake. The myth is therefore true for such diets but not for intermittent fasting. Leonnie Heilbronn and colleagues investigated the effects of alternate-day fasting on different factors, energy metabolism included. In all the 16 nonobese participants, the resting metabolic rate did not change (Heilbronn et al., 2005).

5. **Myth:** Fasting depletes your energy because we all need food to survive.

   Facts: This would be true if the fasting was going to be continuous and prolonged. Otherwise, intermittent fasting involves scheduled fasting hours, followed by "meal times," so there is no way you are going to run out of energy. Besides, you might not be eating, but your body always has some fat reserves of energy that it uses when you're fasting, no matter how lean you might be. Moreover, when you eat, blood flow becomes more directed to the digestive system, as compared to the muscles. Therefore, when you fast, blood flow is directed to other parts of the body more, including the muscles. This is the reason why some feel more energetic when they exercise without eating.

6. **Myth:** You cannot fast and drink water at the same time.

   Facts: Fasting has a diuretic effect. This means that it assists your body to get rid of sodium dissolved in water and releases these as urine (Stanto, n.d). Since sodium is removed from the blood while it is dissolved in water, this has an impact of lowering your blood pressure. The best you can do, for the sake of your health, is to drink water so that you prevent the dangerous effects that accompany dehydration.

Chapter 2: Am I Overweight?

When weight is measured in relation to one's height and compared against a given standard, one can determine whether they are overweight. In this regard, one is overweight when the relationship between their weight and height falls below the standards that are already available in literature. This measure of the relationship between weight and height is commonly referred to as the body mass index (BMI).

Since the parameters for measuring the BMI are weight and height, the only parameter that you can alter to change your BMI is weight. However, there is often a misconception that being overweight is only a factor of too much fat, which is not always the case. Sometimes, one can be overweight due to accumulation of lean muscle, especially those who do strenuous exercises. This implies that even without too much fat, one can have a larger weight as compared to others of the same height as them. Having said that, one can be overweight but not fat at the same time.

Another question that comes to play is, "Is being overweight the same as being obese?" As highlighted earlier, one can be overweight with or without fat. On the contrary, obesity is measured with respect to how much body fat one has. One is obese when the amount of body fat in their body is excessive in reference to their lean body mass. This means that there is too much fat as compared to the body height, and again, this is measured with respect to given standards. Being overweight and obese are only differentiated in terms of fat, which is difficult to analyze. Therefore, both of them are measured as the BMI.

Find Out if You Are Overweight

The BMI method is widely accepted, but there are other ways through which you can determine if you are overweight. This is because there are many other factors that come into play, making it difficult to just confine the analysis of one's overweight status to current weight and height only. In this section, we are going to explore different ways through which you can determine your weight status.

Calculate Your BMI

Before you calculate your BMI, you should know the general standards that help you to categorize your weight as normal, underweight, overweight, or obese. The National Health Institute (NHI) gives the following ranges:

- One is obese when their BMI is over 30.
- When the BMI is between 25 and 29.9, one is overweight.
- A BMI of between 18.5 and 24.9 is reflective of an ideal weight.

- One is considered to be underweight when the BMI is below 18.5.

Now that you have this information in your hands, you can go ahead and calculate your BMI. You can use the BMI calculator, which can calculate your BMI upon providing the details of your current weight and height. The BMI calculator also classifies your results according to the ranges provided by the NHI. You can also calculate your BMI on your own using any of the formulas below (Hazell, 2019):

- BMI = weight (kilograms) / [height (meters)]^2

- BMI = 703 x weight (pounds) / [height (inches]^2

Calculate Your Waist to Height Ratio

Ideally, your waist measurement should be less than half your height. When that is the case, one is considered to not be overweight. To calculate your waist to height ratio, simply divide your waist measurement with your height (both in inches or centimeters). When the result that you get is equal or less than 0.5, it is more likely that you are neither overweight nor obese. Ideally, men should have a waist size that is less than 40 inches, while women's waist size should not surpass 35 inches (Brazier, 2020).

This method of checking one's weight status can be a good screening tool for diseases such as diabetes, heart attacks, high blood pressure, and strokes. This is because fat that accumulates on the waist area can negatively affect the liver, heart, and kidneys. However, just like the BMI method, the waist-to-height-ratio method has its own flaws. It overlooks the need to consider hip size and height in determining an ideal weight.

Calculate Body Fat Percentage

This method describes a person's ideal body weight in terms of one's total fat, which includes essential and storage fat. **Storage fat** is the form in which energy is stored for use during times of stress and energy depletion. It is also the type of fat that covers internal organs, to protect them from physical damage. **Essential fat** is required by the body for survival since it is involved in the body's functions. The American Council on Exercise stipulated that the essential fat amounts should be between 10 and 13%, while those for men should be between 2 and 4%.

To calculate your body fat percentage, use the following formula:

Body fat percentage = (Your total fat weight) divided by (Your total weight)

There are various techniques that can be used to measure your body fat. These include:

- **The skinfold measurement:** This involves pinching a part of your skin using calipers. The skinfold measurement can be done on the upper arm for women, chest for men, as well as the thighs and abdomen for both men and women.

- **Bioelectrical impedance analysis**: The basis for this method is that body composition is determined by measuring the rate at which an electrical current moves through the body. The determination of body fat is based on the principle that movement of the electric current across fats is slower as compared to nonfat regions of the body. Therefore, the fat is estimated by measuring the difference in the rate at which the electric current moves between fatty and nonfat areas of the body (Frey, 2016).

- **Air densitometry:** As you might be aware by now, the human body can be partitioned into two sections: the fat and the nonfat sections. Each compartment has its own density, with the fat having lower density than the fat-free regions. The application of air densitometry in measuring the amount of body fat is based on the assumption that the density of the fat-free parts of the body is relatively the same between individuals, such that the only difference becomes the fat density. Therefore, when your body is compared to the standards, the only variation that is estimated is the amount of fat.

- **Hydrostatic weighing:** This method of measuring body weight is considered to be one of the most accurate techniques for estimating body fat weight. It involves measuring your weight while you are submerged under water using an underwater scale. Your underwater weight is then compared to your land weight, which will have been measured prior to carrying out the underwater weighing procedure. These measurements are necessary for determining your body density, which will in turn be used to estimate your body fat. The principle for this method lies in the fact that fat is lighter than muscles and bones. Therefore, when your underwater weight is relatively lower than your land weight, your body fat percentage is higher. The opposite of this is also true (Yetman, 2020).

- **Computerized Tomography (CT) or Magnetic Resonance Imaging (MRI) Scans:** These are the most accurate techniques for determining body weight, but they can only be conducted by trained specialists. Moreover, the equipment that is used is very expensive and often set aside for research purposes. Using these scans, specialists can view three-dimensional images that show your bones, tissues, and body fat.

Calculate Waist-to-Hip Ratio

This technique compares the size of your waist to that of your hips. If the waist measurement is relatively higher in relation to the hip measurement, it implies that you are overweight, and vice versa. To measure your waist-to-hip ratio, begin by measuring the narrowest part of your waist. Usually, this is just above the belly button. After that, measure the widest part of your hip area. Divide the waist measurement by the hip measurement. Suppose your waist measurement is 30 inches and the hip one is 40, dividing 30 by 40 will give you 0.75 as your waist-to-hip ratio. For males, the ideal waist-to-hip ratio should be below 0.9, while it should be below 0.8 in females. Men with a waist-to-hip ratio above 1.0 are more likely to be overweight, just like the females whose values are above 0.9.

Factors Affecting Your Weight

Body weight is affected by various factors, some of which you might have already noticed as we discussed various techniques for determining whether you are overweight or not. Height, waist size, and hip size are some of the factors that we have already discussed. There are many other factors that come into play, though different weight assessing methods tend to downplay them. We will explore some of such factors in this section. I have classified these factors as either natural or unnatural factors.

Natural Factors

These are factors that influence your weight without your input. No matter how much you try to avoid them, they tend to override your will and efforts. Learn more about these factors in this section.

Age: For most people, ageing positively correlates with weight gain. As they get older, they tend to gain more weight. Usually, weight gain begins during puberty and continues as one gets older, even up through your sixties. Males seem to gain more weight until they are around 55, while females continue still gaining weight up to age 65. Sometimes, the weight gain that couples with age is due to hormonal changes. For example, the increase in weight in men as they age may be due to the progressive drop in testosterone levels. Generally, body fat increases after people reach the age of 30. While these are natural changes that you cannot avoid, you can make efforts to reduce or delay them. Lifestyle changes such as healthy eating and exercising can be of great help.

Genetic factors: Sometimes, obesity and overweight conditions tend to run through generations within the same families. The only way this is possible is through passing on of genes from one generation to the other. The extent to which genes contribute to weight gain varies between individuals. In some people, the genetic effects on weight may be as small as 25%, while they can be as high as 80% in other people. The role of genes in aiding weight gain includes affecting metabolism, appetite, food cravings, and the sense of fullness.

Unnatural Factors

These are the factors that you can alter. In fact, they depend on what you do, think, and believe.

Physical activity: You can choose whether to exercise or not, but the truth of the matter is that your choice affects your body weight. When you lack physical activity, especially when your eating habits are not monitored, there is an increased tendency to gain weight. Exercise helps to burn up extra calories that would otherwise be converted to fat, as long as they are available in the body.

Lifestyles: Sedentary lifestyles are supportive of weight gain. The same applies to eating patterns where no efforts are made to reduce the accumulation of fat. For example, intermittent fasting trims down the probability of amassing fat by giving the body more time to process and utilize the calories that you have eaten. Sometimes, the problem is not even in the food itself but in the preparation methods. Frying and grilling methods of food preparation lead to higher calorie intake. Greater orientation toward diets that are rich in salt, fat, and added sugars plays a huge role in aiding weight gain.

Inadequate sleep: People who sleep less gain more weight because they tend to snack more due to increased eating opportunities. Inadequate sleep also affects the body's metabolism by slowing it down. When metabolism is low, especially for a long time, the body will adjust to using lower amounts of energy to keep its functions running, but that also means that it will store more energy in the form of fats. In the first chapter of this book, we discussed the involvement of the hormones ghrelin and leptin in aiding weight gain as a result of lack of enough sleep. It is recommended that teenagers between 13 and 18 years of age should sleep for at least 8 to 10 hours, adults between 18 and 64 should get at least 7 to 9 hours of sleep, and seniors aged above 64 require 7 or 8 hours of sleep each day.

Medications: Some medications have been linked with weight gain as one of their side effects. While such medication does not impact your willpower, they achieve weight gain by increasing your appetite or reducing the rate at which your metabolism takes place. Examples of medications that enhance weight gain are antipsychotics, antidepressants, and diabetes medications (Corell et al., 2011; McFarlane, 2009; Patten et al., 2011).

Weighing Tips

I will close this chapter by giving you some tips on how you can get the best out of weighing yourself, as well as getting other measurements like waist size. This is important considering that there is no way you are going to be able to keep track of whether you are becoming overweight except by taking one measurement or the other. Maya Angelou once said, "When you know better, you do better." Knowing your weight is the foundation for understanding the need to alter your lifestyle, mindset, eating habits, and many other things. It may even help you to make better decisions in light of the schedules that you should choose for your intermittent fasting, as well as the type of diet to settle for.

Weighing once a week is good enough: It sometimes happens that you may become obsessed with stepping onto the scale every now and then, but believe me, that is not a healthy idea. It will only create more anxiety and possibly stress, especially when the numbers that you see on the scale are not the ones that you like. You might even expose yourself to emotional eating in the process. Checking your weight on the scale one time every week is a great and healthy idea. Choose the same time and day of the week to ensure that your measurements and comparisons are more accurate.

Weigh yourself first thing in the morning: Weigh yourself before you eat or drink anything for best results. This is why the morning for your "weighing day" is the best. The food and drink that you eat before you weigh yourself add to the weight results that are shown on the scale. This gives an incorrect picture of your weight because the food is not yet part of your body. It is the same as weighing yourself while carrying the food in your hands.

Standardize your procedures: The variables that you measure should be the same, each time. If you are measuring your waist size, be sure to measure along the same region every time you do so. Do you measure yourself, or do you let someone measure you? Whatever the case might be, you get the most constant results when the same person takes the measurements.

Check how your clothes fit: Checking for the looseness or tightness of your clothes can be a great way to monitor your weight. This may even give you a more accurate estimation of whether you are gaining fat or losing it. When you lose fat, it is more likely that your clothes are going to fit more loosely. However, when you get onto the scale, you might realize little or no changes on the weight in terms of numbers. This might be because the scale does not necessarily measure fat gain or loss, so even when you lose fat and gain muscle, the scale reflects bigger numbers. On the other hand, losing fat and gaining more muscle makes you look more slender, hence the looseness in fitting clothes.

Chapter 3: Why Should I Start Intermittent Fasting?

In Chapter 1, we explored some of the myths that are circulating around social media about intermittent fasting. One of the myths that I did no mention is that "intermittent fasting has no benefits at all." Other opinions about intermittent fasting suggest that the practice will just be one more fad diet. For this reason, this chapter is dedicated to providing you with the facts that nullify such myths and opinions. It also gives you science-based evidence that supports the various benefits of intermittent fasting. By the end of this chapter, you should be enlightened about what intermittent fasting can do for you and why you should consider giving a thought and then a try.

What's in It for You?

What are the benefits of intermittent fasting? This section will answer this question by touring you through some of the benefits that come with practising intermittent fasting.

Trim Down Pounds

Intermittent fasting helps you to lose weight, if you desire to. However, you have to choose the type of intermittent fasting that suits this need. Opting for an intermittent fasting method that involves less than 10 hours of fasting may not be a very good idea in this case. This is because it takes about 10 to 12 hours for the body to use up its glycogen stores in the liver, and only then can it turn the fat stores. Having said this, an intermittent fasting pattern which involves 16 hours of fasting will be ideal for a person who wants to lose weight. By breaking down the fats to obtain energy, the fatty reserves that add to your weight are removed from your body. This progressively reduces your weight, especially when it is done with consistency over time. Commitment is key.

The other way through which intermittent fasting contributes to your weight loss endeavors is by reducing your calorie consumption. This, however, only works when you do not eat to compensate for the meals that you did not eat. This way, the meals that you will have missed are a good enough reduction on the total number of calories that you will have consumed the whole day, if you had not skipped any meals. Reducing calorie intake implies that there will be fewer calories available for conversion to storage fat. Most of the calories will either be used by the body immediately after absorption into the bloodstream, or they will be converted to glycogen stores in the liver and muscles. That having been said, intermittent fasting is not an abrupt way to lose weight but still works in the long run.

A review that was done to investigate the effects of intermittent fasting on weight and other biomarkers concluded that the practice is effective in reducing weight (Ganesan et al., 2018). Another study also reported that intermittent fasting can successfully improve the lipid profile in all people by reducing low density lipoproteins (LDL), triglycerides, and total cholesterol, while it increases the concentrations of high density lipoproteins (HDL) (Santos & Macedo, 2018). The estimated rate at which weight is lost with intermittent fasting is 0.55 to 1.65 pounds (0.25 to 0.75 kilograms) in one week (Gunnars, 2020).

Prevent Some Diseases

The risk of some diseases is reduced when one practices intermittent fasting. By virtue of its efficacy in reducing body weight, intermittent fasting lowers the risk of **type 2 diabetes,** a condition in which the body either fails to produce its own insulin or the body cells resist the insulin that is produced by the body. Either way, body cells are not able to take up glucose, making it accumulate in the bloodstream. Weight loss also reduces the risk of **cardiovascular ailments** by attending to one's heart health. Intermittent fasting reduces blood pressure, thereby further improving heart health. Experiments that were done using animal models showed cardiovascular-promoting effects such as an improved heart rate and reduced levels of blood cholesterol (Aly, 2014).

Reduces Inflammation and Oxidative Stress

Oxidative stress is usually a contributing factor to the progression of many chronic diseases, as well as aging. The biological processes of the body naturally release some unstable, oxidative radicals. Normally, the body has a robust antioxidant system which is responsible for continually removing the oxidative radicals because they are quite destructive if they remain present in the body. However, sometimes the rate at which the free radicals are produced surpasses the rate at which they are removed by the body's antioxidant system, and this causes oxidative stress in the body. Oxidative stress is associated with conditions such as Parkinson's disease and Alzheimer's disease, both of which are linked to the brain. It also causes cardiovascular disorders.

Inflammation is another root cause of many diseases, including arthritis, cancers, stomach ulcers, and bowel diseases like Crohn's diseases. Interestingly, there are studies which support the fact that intermittent fasting counters inflammation triggers, preventing such a wide array of diseases from progressing (Johnson et al., 2007; Faris et al., 2007).

Affects Cellular, Genetic, and Hormonal Function

When you do intermittent fasting, your body responds by making some changes to the way cells, genes, and hormones function. Here are some of the changes that take place during the fasting period of your intermittent fasting:

- **Autophagy:** Intermittent fasting promotes autophagy, which is an important homeostatic process which results in the degradation of cellular components that need to be removed from cells (Alirezaei et al., 2010). This includes removal of waste material from ells. This and cellular repair functions enhance the better functioning of the body's cells. Food restriction methods, including intermittent fasting, upregulate autophagy in the liver and other body organs but not the brain.
- **Insulin hormone levels:** One study revealed that one of the many changes that occur during fasting is reduction of insulin levels (Heilbronn et al., 2005). When insulin levels are higher in the blood, the body's cells will be continually taking up energy in the form of glucose, so there won't be a need for energy from fat reserves. In other words, higher levels of insulin prevent the breakdown of fats in the body. When insulin levels diminish, lipolysis, which is the breakdown of fats, is triggered.
- **Genes and genetic expression:** A review that was published by Bronwem Martin and colleagues in 2006 reported that intermittent fasting can alter the gene

expression of genes that are associated with aging and the health span of the nervous system. The same study reported that intermittent fasting accesses and affects signaling pathways that are involved in regulating lifespan. This enhances longevity. Intermittent fasting also improves the efficiency of energy use, the body's response to oxidative free radicals, and the way cells respond to stress. This way, the practice shields neurons from damage and degradation by various environmental and genetic factors that would otherwise hasten the process of aging. The effects of intermittent fasting on the nervous system also reduce the risk of diseases such as Alzheimer's and Parkinson's disease (Martin et al., 2006).

Brain Health Is Improved

The health of the brain is often dependent on the health of other organs of the body. This is because the functionality of all the other parts of the body is connected to the brain in one way or the other. In fact, most of the body's processes are regulated by the various parts of the brain.

The role of intermittent fasting in improving the healthy functioning of other body processes, including heart health and the nervous system, impacts the health of the brain. The reduction of blood sugar levels, free oxidative radicals, and inflammation promotes a healthier brain (Gunnars, 2016).

A study that investigated the effects of food restriction on rats showed that the growth of new neurons increased upon restricting food intake (Lee et al., 2000). Increased expression of Brain-Derived Neurotrophic Factor (BDNF) was also reported in the same study. The BDNF is the major molecule involved in enhancing changes that are associated with memory and learning. When people learn new things, new connections take place between neurons, resulting in changes in the nervous system as a whole. Therefore, by enhancing the expression of BDNF, intermittent fasting builds up the learning capacity and memory of an individual.

A reduced mortality rate from ischemic stroke was discovered in a study that was done using mice, and the results were attributed to intermittent fasting (Arumugam et al., 2010). Ischemic stroke is a type of stroke that results from the blockage of the artery that takes blood to the brain. The brain is deprived of blood and oxygen, a state which causes death of brain cells. By improving the flow of blood through all blood vessels, intermittent fasting is an effective tool in trimming down the risk of ischemic stroke.

Boosts Metabolism

If fasting is stretched over long periods, the rate at which metabolism takes place reduces. On the other hand, shorter periods of fasting boost your metabolism. One of the scientific studies that support this notion reported that the metabolism of 11 male participants who underwent fasting for three days increased by 14% (Zaunar et al., 2000). This is a remarkable improvement. Scientists suggest that such an increase in the rate of metabolism might be due to an increased secretion of epinephrine.

Intermittent Fasting and Teenagers

Many concerns have been aired by parents and other guardians about whether teenagers should engage in intermittent fasting. Despite the various reasons that some give in support of the notion that teenagers should not do intermittent fasting, I beg to differ. Having said that, I support the idea that intermittent fasting is equally good for teenagers as it is for adults. After all, there is never a completely good way of monitoring your eating patterns; each method has its own flaws. Everything boils down to an individual's choice with regards to the method of monitoring food intake. To ease your decision-making process, I will highlight some of the reasons why I recommend intermittent fasting for teenagers.

The type of intermittent fasting matters: It is well understood that teenagers are in a period of rapid growth, and their body cells require as much nourishment from food as possible. However, it is also important to note that not all types of intermittent fasting affect the growth needed by teenagers. Intermittent fasting may only become a concern to teenagers when the fasting period stretches to 20 hours and beyond. Shorter periods of fasting will not lead to a starvation mode, and less physical stress will have been realized from not eating food. In fact, the body only enters starvation mode after 72 hours without food. This is the time when the body turns to the muscle for energy, having depleted all other sources—that is, the glycogen stores in the liver and the fat stores. Only then, can intermittent fasting be detrimental to teens who are experiencing a growth spurt. Otherwise, teenagers can partake in intermittent fasting.

Good nutrition is a concern for all people: Even without intermittent fasting, all people, including teenagers, require nutrient-dense food to nourish their body and stay healthy. Therefore, intermittent fasting works well for both teenagers and adults if, after the fast, they eat a balanced diet with relatively all nutrients in their right quantities. For teenagers, more emphasis should be put on foods that enhance growth. For example, zinc is important for growth, and its deficiency can lead to stunted growth. Therefore, intermittent fasting has no detrimental effects on the growth and development of teenagers unless they do not eat foods that support and enhance growth during the periods when they are not fasting.

Some teenagers have some fat to lose: As highlighted earlier, intermittent fasting can aid weight loss. There are greater chances that kids who suffer from obesity in their teenage years will also suffer from it as adults. Attending to your body and staying fit as a teenager is a great way to avoid the risk of obesity when you become an adult. Getting yourself into the habit of intermittent fasting at a young age makes it less difficult to maintain, even as an adult. Besides, the effects of accumulating fat in your body are way too detrimental, even in the long run, as compared to the effort that you put in enhancing calorie deficit through fasting.

Human growth hormone (HGH) levels rise during fasting: One of the reasons that teenagers grow at a faster rate is due the doubled production of HGH at puberty. This hormone drops as soon as the puberty stage is over. Interestingly, levels of HGH rise during intermittent fasting (Ho et al., 1988). This could imply that growth is enhanced rather than compromised, as long as your nutrient requirements are being met at the same time.

Intermittent fasting has health benefits: The health benefits that are associated with intermittent fasting are good for teenagers, in the same way that they are to adults. Teenagers also need to reduce the risk of cardiovascular diseases, some cancers, and neurodegenerative diseases. They even need neuroplasticity, which enhances learning and memory, maybe even more than the adults do because the teenagers are at a stage where they learn a lot of new things at the same time.

Intermittent Fasting and Senior Adults

There is no doubt that intermittent fasting works well in improving your health, as exhibited by the wide array of benefits that are associated with the practice. However, some are skeptical about whether the practice is safe for the elderly.

Intermittent fasting is safe for the elderly. Besides, as people age, they are less able to engage in strenuous physical activity as they used to do.

In addition to benefits that have already been discussed in this chapter, there are other benefits that are associated with older age, that senior adults can take advantage of by practising intermittent fasting. We will explore some of these additional benefits in this section.

Memory and cognitive acumen: As people age, their memory and cognitive abilities progressively decline. It becomes more and more difficult to remember the things that they would normally remember in their younger ages. Evidence from studies shows that intermittent fasting enhances working, associative, and spatial memory and reduces the risk of cognitive decline (Li et al., 2013; Shin et al., 2018). While memory and cognitive decline are naturally part of ageing, the rate at which they occur can be reduced by intermittent fasting.

Balance and coordination: Aging is also associated with loss of balance and coordination. Studies on animal models showed that intermittent fasting improves balance and coordination, and this can be useful to senior citizens (Ktetzschmer, 2020).

Chapter 4: Begin the Process and Make It Work

Intermittent fasting goes hand-in-hand with a low-carb diet because it cuts down on the carbohydrates that you consume over time. Both low-carbohydrate diets and intermittent fasting can help you to break down the stored fat that would otherwise not be used up as long as there are other sources of food in the body.

We explored the different benefits that are associated with intermittent fasting. You might have realized that intermittent fasting is the answer to some of the food-associated problems that you have been facing. In that case, one or more benefits of intermittent fasting could be your motivation to start the process. This chapter is dedicated to helping you to embark on your LCIF journey.

Motivate Yourself

The decision to do LCIF could be one of the best decisions that you make in your life because it concerns your health. However, it does not come on a silver platter; you work for it. Starting the journey is not an easy task but not an impossible one, though. As long as it is not impossible, then there is a way to make it happen. It starts with motivating yourself. In this section, I have compiled some tips that can help you to get started with LCIF.

Why Is LCIF Important?

One of the best motivations that you can give yourself is identifying the reason why you think the LCIF combination is the one for you. There is no point in embarking on a shift from your normal eating patterns just for the sake for it. There must be one or more reasons attached to your decision. Is it because you want to watch your weight? Do you even want to reduce the weight? Are your concerns more on health? Probably, the work that you do needs a lot of focus and memory, and you want to keep your brain healthy and up for the task. It could be that you are approaching an older age, and you are worried about the cognitive decline that is associated with ageing. You might have other underlying conditions such as diabetes and high blood pressure that can have an impact on the functioning capacities of the brain. It could be that you just want to improve your metabolism and feel more energetic.

Whatever your reason might be, it can be a great motivation, if you let it. Whenever you feel skeptical about the fact that you won't be eating food as you used to, just think about why you decided to do LCIF in the first place. Tell yourself, "I have to drop some pounds within the next five months," if that suits you. You will be surprised at how much this will sharpen your focus on your LCIF procedures.

Feed Yourself With the Right Information

Sometimes, motivation depends on what you see, hear, or read. Due to technology, information has become ubiquitous, and finding the right information in such a large pool can be difficult. However, if you are able to do it, the motivation that you get from it may be just what you need to get yourself started.

Watch some videos, read some blogs, and derive your motivation from other people's stories. There are many testimonies out there about intermittent fasting or the low-carbohydrate diet, but unless you search for them, you can't benefit from them. Find out how other people survived the hurdles that are involved in starting intermittent fasting. How did they go about the discouragement that comes from friends, relatives, and family concerning the choice to do LCIF? Learn from experts and others who have traveled the journey before. If they could do it, then so can you!

Deal With Your Mindset

Your mindset has everything to do with your motivation to take up LCIF. When you do something that your mind does not approve of, you might not make it in the long run, that is if you would have started it anyway. Your mindset can be the culprit to stop you from engaging in LCIF. For example, if you see intermittent fasting and low-carbohydrate diets as a form of punishment for, say, overeating and being overweight, you are less likely to enjoy any of the process. You will be less motivated to start, let alone continue over time.

What you need is a mind shift. Do not connect your past mistakes with your decision to do LCIF, unless you look at your past blunders in a way that they motivate you not to repeat them. For instance, you might say, "I do not want to eat unnecessarily like I did for the past two years, otherwise I will become overweight again." This is different from saying, "If I hadn't eaten too much for the past two years, my weight would have been okay, and I wouldn't have to do this LCIF." Can you see that the first example is more motivating than the second one?

Think of the Possible End

If you have never engaged in any form of fasting before, LCIF might sound very difficult. This might cause you to hesitate taking it up. In such cases, picturing the end that you expect might be a great strategy. Suppose that you want to do LCIF because you want to lose weight. Visualizing yourself having achieved your target weight and imagining the good feelings that this will bring you can get you started. You will start LCIF with the motivation of wanting to be the person that you visualize yourself to be.

Set Your Goals

Success in any endeavor is more certain when you are able to sit down and put your goals in place. This might even involve writing them down. Writing your goals helps to keep your motivation lit. There are three goals that will make LCIF a success for you and I will discuss these in this section.

1. Stopping your previous eating patterns

The first goal, as far as starting LCIF is concerned, is to realize that you need to stop the way you have been eating, especially if it wasn't healthy. Identify what you did not like about your previous eating patterns, as compared to what you know about LCIF. See the benefits of LCIF that you would miss by continuing with your unhealthy eating patterns.

There are many diets that encourage eating patterns that are contrary to what is recommended through LCIF. For example, if you were used to the idea that missing your breakfast makes you less energetic for the rest of your day, that would mean that you had to eat something first thing every morning. Some diet regimens recommend that you eat small but frequent meals throughout the day for you to lose weight and stay healthy. All these notions contradict with how LCIF works. Therefore, once you decide that you want to take up LCIF, you should make a bold decision to wave goodbye to any other patterns of eating that are not in line with the practice. When this goal is in place, then you can set the next goal.

2. Starting LCIF

Starting LCIF is a goal on its own. This will require you to choose the days that you want to be fasting. There are different types of intermittent fasting. Their difference is mainly in the length of the fasting periods. The length of your fasting period is dependent on various aspects, including the reasons why you are doing intermittent fasting. We will discuss more about the variations of intermittent fasting in the next chapter. However, for now, I recommend that you choose the intermittent fasting pattern that is feasible for you, to reduce the probability of giving up.

3. Making LCIF Part of Your Lifestyle

The long-term benefits of LCIF are better realized when you incorporate the eating pattern into your lifestyle. To do this, make living a "healthy lifestyle" the major reason why you are following the LCIF pattern. Most of the other benefits that you can think of emanate from this major goal, yet making them your main goal, will give you an endpoint for your LCIF eating pattern. For instance, you eat the "LCIF way" in order to lose 20 pounds of weight. Once you achieve that, you will feel that you don't need to fast anymore because you got what you wanted. On the contrary—when your goal is "being healthy," this is a lifetime endeavor. As you work toward it every day, you will achieve all the other subgoals like weight loss, reducing risks of diseases, and enhancing cognitive acumen. In fact, it is best to call these subgoals your objectives because they feed to the main goal.

Ask Your Questions

To better prepare you to start intermittent fasting, I would like to give you some tips on how to get started with intermittent fasting. To accomplish this, I have set aside this section to answer some of the questions that you might have concerning LCIF. Once your questions are cleared up, you can go ahead and enjoy your healthy lifestyle through LCIF.

What is the history of intermittent fasting?

People who lived on this earth a long time ago were hunter-gatherers. It was not always obvious that they would find food to eat each day. They would, therefore, go for days without finding something to eat. That was a form of fasting. As time elapsed, people began to fast willingly, mainly for religious purposes. The concept of intermittent fasting was introduced about a decade ago, but it gained popularity in 2012 when the documentary titled *"Eat, Fast, and Live Longer"* was aired (Lawler, 2020).

Skipping meals is unusual to me. Won't I feel hungry?

If you have been having frequent meals, your body will have become accustomed to your eating patterns. Just before the time that you usually eat, your body prepares itself to receive some food by, for example, beginning the secretion of insulin to regulate the expected surges in blood glucose.

It will take your body some time to adjust to your newly adopted way of eating. In the initial days, you might find it more difficult to miss the meals that you used to eat. Your body will be reminding you that you have to eat. However, with focus and endurance, your body will adjust and get used to taking fewer meals in a day.

The same applies as you cut down on the carbohydrate levels that you consume during each meal. If you were used to eating large amounts of carbohydrates, your body will also take its time to adjust and manage the fewer calories that you will be providing it with. You should also take note of the fact that if you are overweight, you might find it more difficult to switch to LCIF because overweight people tend to eat more. However, as I mentioned earlier, being delayed is not being denied. No matter how much time it might take, you can do it.

Can I have some fruits in between meals during intermittent fasting?

Intermittent fasting involves two windows: the fasting and the feasting windows. During the fasting period, you should not eat food. Once you are in the feasting window, you can eat as much as you want. Whether you want to have two or three meals during the fasting period is a matter of choice.

My understanding is that working out requires energy. Will I still be able to work out while I fast at the same time?

Surprisingly, results from studies suggest that it is even better for you to work out without having a preworkout meal (van Proeyen et al., 2011). When you work out after eating, your body will use the carbohydrates from your meal to provide the energy required by the muscle cells. In the event that you did not eat, the muscles cells turn to the fat reserves in your body for energy. Mind you, everyone has fat reserves, even the leanest person. So, yes, you will be able to simultaneously work out and fast.

Which time of the day is best for me to fast?

It is difficult to pinpoint the time of the day that you must fast. However, an important fact that might help you to decide is that your body becomes more insulin resistant as the day progresses. This implies that you are less insulin resistant during the early hours of the day, as compared to the late hours. Based on this fact, it might be advisable that you eat your food earlier in the day when it can be better metabolized. You can then start your fast hours before your sleeping time (Jarreau, 2018). This way, you give your body food during the time when it can efficiently metabolize it and fast when the efficiency to deal with nutrients is less.

How much food should I consume during the "feasting period" of my fast?

Generally, how much you should eat when you are fasting intermittently depends on yourself and your objectives. Remember, we said that the main goal is to stay healthy. If losing weight is your objective, then you need to trim down how much you eat. While most diet regimens suggest that you should drastically cut down on all food components, the LCIF recommends that you monitor the amount of carbohydrates that you eat. If your objective is not to lose weight, you need to balance the protein, fat, vitamin, and mineral sources to keep your eating healthy. Processed food is not a good option, though. One other thing—LCIF will not change unhealthy food to become healthy. If you eat unhealthy food during your feasting window, its negative effects may equally affect you.

Are there any side effects that I should expect from intermittent fasting?

Like any eating protocol, intermittent fasting has its own side effects that you may need to be aware of before you start. Most of the side effects of intermittent fasting are due to being unused to the practice. For example, some may experience nausea, migraines, insomnia, and dizziness. You might also feel hungry and less energetic during the fasting period. Some females experience irregularities in their menstrual cycle. However, it is important that you see the doctor if you miss your menstruation period for three months or more in a row.

Chapter 5: Intermittent Fasting Variation

Intermittent fasting can be done in different ways depending on the preferences that people have. While the concept of the practice is the same, the main difference is in the number of hours for the fasting and the feasting windows. In some cases, the length of the fasting and feasting periods might be the same, but individuals choose what time of the day the feasting window begins or ends. Such preferences are influenced by various factors which include work schedules, daily routines, family rules, cultures, climates, and religious affiliations. This implies that the decision to start intermittent fasting is beyond the thought of just admiring someone who does it or looking at the benefits. While these are also important factors, it is even more important that you consider different factors for you to come up with the fasting variation and method that suits you. In this chapter, we will delve more into the different variations of intermittent fasting. Hopefully, you choose your best fit!

Major Types of Intermittent Fasting

According to the *Merriam-Webster* dictionary, the term "intermittent" means "coming and going at intervals." This implies that there is a break in continuity. In the context of intermittent fasting, the term describes the alternating intervals of fasting and eating. This can be done in different ways. The many major types of intermittent fasting that exist will be explained in this section.

Weekly Intermittent Fasting

In this type of fasting, you only spend the day without eating once in a week. You choose one day that you would like to fast, while you eat the rest of the days of the week. For example, you might decide to stop eating, say, on Monday afternoon. You sleep without eating and wake up the next day, which is Tuesday morning. You may then start eating on Tuesday afternoon (Clear, 2012).

Weekly fasting can help you to overcome the fears that are associated with fasting. For instance, after successfully completing a day, you may realize that fasting is possible and that you don't die when you fast. It is, however, unlikely that one can lose weight through this type of intermittent fasting because they are eating most of the time. Ideally, you would be missing two meals in a week. The calorie intake does not reduce, yet little will be done to burn the fat stores in the body. The greater possibility is that weight might even increase. However, there are many other benefits that one enjoys as a result of this fasting. It is reported that the body actually functions better when you are fasting. Your alertness, cognitive acumen, memory, and learning are all better when the body is in the fasting state (Wnuk, 2018).

Alternate-Day Intermittent Fasting

Alternate-day intermittent fasting is more frequent than the weekly variation. You fast one day (except for the night) and eat the next day. For instance, suppose it's a Wednesday and you eat your last meal at 7:00 p.m. That is when your fasting will begin, and you will spend the whole of the next day without eating. Your next meal would be at 7:00 p.m. on Thursday. You will freely eat for the whole of the next Friday until 7:00 p.m., which is when the fasting that will end Saturday will start. Simply said, your fasting and eating will take place in alternating periods of 24 hours for each window.

While there is a lot of research that is going on concerning the alternate-day fasting method, it is unfortunate that this type of fasting is the most unpopular. It is more theoretical than it is practical. However, this type of fasting is more beneficial than the weekly type of fasting because the fasting windows are longer.

Alternating-Hours Intermittent Fasting

Some people prefer to fast continually for some days, while they monitor the number of hours that they eat and those that they do not eat. Such type of fasting cannot be described as weekly fasting because the fasting is done more than once a week. On the other hand, it's not alternate-day fasting because fasting can be done every other day, even on consecutive days.

In this book, we are going to focus more on the intermittent hours type of fasting. Therefore, all the types of fasting that are going to be explored in this section are variations of the type of fasting that can be done every day. These include the 12-hour, 14-hour , and 16-hour types of fasting.

The 10-Hour Fasting Variation

The lowest number of hours that one can fast is 10 hours. This is because fasting is not done just for the sake of it; there has to be expected results. Studies show that the benefits of fasting begin to be evident when the fasting window is 10 hours and above. It is reported that fasting periods between 10 and 16 hours encourage the body to break down fats in order to get energy from them (Collier, 2010). This is because the glycogen stores in the liver will have been exhausted and so the body turns to its fat stores.

The 10-hour fasting method is also great for beginners and teenagers. The eating window lasts for 14 hours, while the fasting stretches for only 10 hours. This type of fasting does not cause you to lose much in terms of calories, and this makes it a great option for teenagers, who are experiencing growth spurts. For fasting amateurs, the 10-hour fasting method can be a good training ground as far as fasting is concerned. There is a beginning to everything. Besides, the journey of a thousand miles begins with a single step. Once you are acquainted with the 10-hr fasting routine, you can upgrade to more fasting hours for more benefits.

Some experts, however, recommend more hours of fasting for better effects, especially on metabolism and other body functions. Just in the same way that sleep rejuvenates the body and makes it more energetic, fasting also promotes similar results. This is because when you constantly eat, your cells and the rest of the body are constantly busy with processes such as digestion, absorption, assimilation, and relevant nervous transmission. Hours of not eating gives the body some rest, and this enhances its functions.

How can you do the 10-hour fasting method? You can start fasting at 8:00 p.m. and end your fasting at 6:00 a.m. the next day if you prefer to fast during your sleeping hours. Alternatively, you can fast from 8:00 a.m. to 6:00 p.m. of the same day if you are more inclined to fasting during the day. Any other choices are acceptable, as long as the fasting period will not be less than the stipulated 10 hours.

The 12-Hour Fasting Variation

In the 12-hour fasting variation, the fasting hours are the same as the feasting hours. You fast for 12 hours and eat for the other 12 hours of the day. This type of intermittent fasting is recommended for beginners who are not yet used to the longer fasting hours.

While it may seem like the fasting and feasting windows are the same for the 12-hour fasting variation, technically it is not true. The fasting period eats into sleeping hours, making it relatively smaller than the eating period. Simply said, most of the fasting is done when you are asleep, so the hours that you consciously fast are fewer. There is even a possibility that the calories that you consume per day may not be significantly reduced. That makes it more comfortable as compared to the other fasting methods.

To begin the 12-hour fasting variation, you need to decide when you prefer to fast. For example, you could decide to stop eating at 7:30 p.m. on a Tuesday, and that would mean that you will start eating again after 12 hours. In other words, you will start eating again at 7:30 a.m. on Wednesday. Incorporating your sleeping hours into the fasting period is probably the easiest way to do this type of intermittent fasting.

The 14-hour Fasting Variation

This is the opposite of the 10-hour fasting routine. Instead of feasting for 14 hours as is the case with the 10-hour fasting methods, the 14-hour fasting regimen is practiced by fasting for 14 hours and feeding for 10 hours. Be sure not to confuse the two.

One of the studies that investigated the effects of the 14-hour fasting method showed that the overweight participants in the study had a 3% weight loss and 4% loss of abdominal visceral fat (Wilkinson et al., 2020). This shows that even 10 hours of eating causes the body to reach out to the fat stores for its energy, hence the significant loss of weight and fat.

It is interesting to note that this type of fasting additionally increases the benefits that intermittent fasting offers to the body. The increased efficiency of the body's metabolic processes ensures that important nutrients are broken down more effectively. Antioxidants that play a crucial role in delaying ageing are released into the bloodstream more efficiently. The natural antioxidants add to the antioxidant system of the body and remove oxygen and nitrogen reactive free radicals that increase the rate at which body cells are damaged. Remember, aging is a natural process that is aided by cell damage.

If you start your fast at 8:00 p.m. on a Monday, then you will break your fast at 10:00 a.m. the next day. After that, your eating spree begins until you begin the other fast at 8:00 p.m. on Tuesday. It is important to note that you choose your fasting hours on your own, depending on what is convenient to you. What is important is to maintain the length of your fasting window.

The 16-hour Fasting Variation

In this type of fasting, you refrain from eating for 16 hours, leaving an eating window of only 8 hours. Because of this fasting and eating pattern, this type of fasting is called the 16-8 method of intermittent fasting. It is alternatively known as the Leangains diet (Leonard, 2020).

In the 16-hour fasting variation, male teenagers and adults fast for 16 hours, while the females fast for 14 hours (Leonard, 2020). "Why should women fast for less hours than men?", you might be wondering. Results from experimental studies have shown that the effects of intermittent fasting are different in males and females. In one study, the researchers observed that three weeks of fasting reduced blood sugar control. These effects were not observed in men who underwent the same period of fasting (Heilbronn et al., 2005).

There have also been reports of changes in the menstrual cycles of women as a result of fasting. The main reason why this occurs is that the bodies of women are structured in such a way that they are affected by extreme limitations in calories. For ovulation to occur, estrogen and the luteinizing hormone should increase in concentration. On the other hand, some studies revealed that the levels of the luteinizing hormone depend on the calorie consumption of females (Loucks et al., 1998). For females whose energy intake is lower than 30 kilocalories per kilogram, there is a risk of having lower concentrations of the luteinizing hormones, thereby affecting menstruation and fertility (Loucks & Thuma, 2003).

To do the 16-8 fasting method, you can eat your last meal at 8:00 p.m. You will then skip breakfast. You will only eat your next meal in the afternoon, around 2:00 p.m., after which the floating window will have started. The effects of reducing the eating window to eight hours was investigated on mice. The study showed that the 16-8 fasting method reduced the risk of diabetes, liver disease, obesity, and inflammation, despite how much was consumed during the eating window (Hatori et al., 2012).

Chapter 6: Eat All You Want Without Gaining Weight

Most diets and weight-managing endeavors are focused on eating less, completely restricting the consumption of some foods and reducing the amounts of the ones that are eaten. In these diets, the focus is more on what to eat than what not to eat. Contrary to these other eating patterns, intermittent fasting focuses more on when to eat than what to eat. In other words, intermittent fasting stipulates the times to eat and not to eat but is not strict on what should be eaten during the eating window. LCIF just encourages people to eat low-carbohydrate foods so that they monitor their calorie intake. It is important to note that there is no complete restriction of carbohydrates, and by the way, you can eat all other foods, without worrying about failing the diet, as long as you eat during the feasting window.

The strength of LCIF is in being faithful to the schedule of your selected type of intermittent fasting, particularly the fasting hours. This is when all the excess calories and fats that have accumulated during the eating window are burned up through the natural processes of the body. The breakdown of fats when the body has exhausted other energy supplies is a natural process, which is only triggered, in this case, by fasting. The fasting session on its own helps you to reduce some unplanned consumption of calories through snacking.

The bottom line is that no matter how much you eat during the feasting window, it is more likely to be exhausted during your next fasting window. This reduces the probability of gaining weight and accumulating visceral fat. Instead, weight is lost, fat is burned, and the desired weight can be maintained without extreme focus on restricting food consumption and altering eating patterns. This chapter concentrates on the eating window of intermittent fasting schedules. How are you supposed to handle this session? Get the answers to some of your questions in this chapter.

What Should I Eat?

My direct answer to this question is, "Eat all you want. You will not gain any weight." Surprised? I knew you would be. Due to the emphasis that most diets and weight loss regimens place on monitoring every little food item that you eat, when people see food, they see ingredients for weight gain. This is why you are more conscious of calorie intake as you eat, more than you are of the benefits that the food has for your body. What happened to that holistic approach to food? Food is supposed to nourish our bodies and eating should be a pleasure, not the other way round.

The best answer to what you should eat can be derived from answering the question, "Why do I need to eat?" Of course, you eat because you are hungry, but there is more beyond that. When you feel hungry, your body is alerting you of the depletion of nutrients in your body. All the processes that take place in your body require one or the other nutrient, which is the reason why you should eat. Now, back to the main question, "What should I eat?" Eat the food that will provide your body with the various nutrients that it needs, in quantities that are not below what the body requires. Consuming the right quantities of nutrients is an ideal situation but is usually not practically feasible. Having said this, I am of the notion that the more nutrients, the better. You won't gain the weight, trust me. The excess nutrients that would have been converted to fat will be burned during your next fasting session.

Let us have a look at some of the nutrients that should be made available to your body through what you eat.

Carbohydrates

Carbohydrates are associated with high calorie content, and that is why many people are "scared" of them. However, the truth of the matter is that your body needs them, and that is why we do not recommend that you completely remove them from your diet. The best that you can do is to lower your consumption but not below the recommended levels. Typically, a meal in the Western diet may contain 250 grams or more of carbohydrates, most of which are refined carbohydrates like sugars. This brings us to yet another question, "How low is a low-carbohydrate diet?"

Dr. Andreas Eenfeldt categorized low-carbohydrate diets into three categories, as follows (Eenfeldt, 2021):

- **Ketogenic low carbohydrates:** This refers to a carbohydrate consumption that amounts to lower than 20 grams per day. This is extremely low in concentration of this important nutrient.
- **Moderate low carbohydrate:** A total of 20 to 50 grams of carbohydrates per day is consumed.
- **Liberal low carbohydrates**: In this case, the daily total for carbohydrate consumption is 50 to 100 grams.

Carbohydrates are the main source of energy for the body. They can be easily broken down and, therefore, can provide the body with quick energy. When the amount of carbohydrates in your diet is reasonably reduced, most of them are used to provide the energy that is required by the body, leaving lesser amounts for conversion to fat. Moreover, more carbohydrates are associated with feeling hungry more frequently, since they are quickly broken down and used for energy. Rice and pasta are the most common sources of high amounts of carbohydrates. Lower carbohydrate amounts can be obtained from eating broccoli, cauliflower, nuts, leafy green vegetables, fish, and fruits.

Proteins

LCIF allows you to eat as much protein as your body requires. Most nutritional organizations recommend a Dietary Reference Intake (DRI) of 0.36 grams per pound, which is equivalent to 0.8 grams per kilogram (Gunners, 2020).

Interpreting these protein dietary requirements means that sedentary men require approximately 56 grams, while women require 46 grams. These are quite generous amounts for a person who is following intermittent fasting. Generally speaking, it simply means eat as much protein as you want!

Most of the molecules that regulate various processes in the body have proteins as their building blocks. Hormones, enzymes, and neurotransmitters are some of the molecules that are made up of proteins. These molecules are degraded daily, and more need to be made by the body. Now, imagine what the situation is like in the body when there is limited consumption of proteins. Some of the foods that are rich in proteins are fish, eggs, beef, and plant products such as beans.

Fats

I am completely aware of the fact that LCIF does not make an unhealthy diet healthier. It simply provides a better way to improve metabolism in the body. This ensures that all nutrients are fully metabolized. As emphasized earlier, intermittent fasting reduces accumulation of fat in the body. Having said this, it is important to understand that the fact you are making efforts to reduce the accumulation of fat does not necessarily imply that you don't need fats in your body.

There are different types of fats that exist, some of which are healthy and required by the body for certain functions in the body. Some body parts are insulated from damage by fats.

Such fats, which include cholesterol, triglycerides, and some essential fatty acids that the body cannot make on its own, support proteins in carrying out their functions by acting as messengers. Imagine how you would store your excess energy for emergencies if you had no fats in your body. Fats are also involved in hormone regulation, brain function, gene regulation, and absorption of vitamins that are fat soluble (Spritzler, 2020).

Various health organizations have been advocating for lower daily fat intake. This has led many people to put all possible effort into eliminating intake of fat. While it is difficult to determine how much fat one should consume, the benefits that you can get from fats are clear evidence that fats are a requirement in your body. However, there are types of fats that are recommended more than others. Generally, you should eat more monounsaturated fats, limit saturated fats, and refrain from trans fats (Madell & Nall, 2020). Food such as avocados and sardines are great sources of recommended fats.

Vitamins and Other Nutrients

What you eat should also contain vitamins and minerals, as well as fiber. All these nutrients contribute to the well-being of the body. Vitamin C is known for its antioxidant properties. Various minerals are involved in bone formation and maintenance. Some such minerals act as cofactors in enzymes that catalyze important reactions in the body. For example, copper and zinc work together with the superoxide dismutase enzyme, which is an antioxidant enzyme.

To obtain much out of food, variety is key. No one food is rich in all nutrients. Therefore, depending on your preferences, availability of the food, and other factors, you can eat a variety of food components.

Get the Body Moving—Exercise

Unrestricted eating, coupled with fasting and a low-carbohydrate diet, works well when you take some time to exercise. An object in motion stays in motion, while an object at rest stays at rest. Exercise and eating patterns are inseparable aspects. In fact, exercising completes the cycle of developing and maintaining a sound body. Exercising is associated with increased willpower toward achieving goals. This is because when you commit yourself to exercising regularly, you develop self-control, which is one of the factors that increase willpower.

Sometimes, people make the effort to start exercising regularly; they pay monthly subscriptions to gyms and purchase some sportswear, but they give up somewhere along the way. I believe that it is easier to give up on hard, strenuous, and complicated exercise than it is for more simple ones. I will suggest some exercises that you can consider doing to keep yourself healthy and how you can fit them into your busy schedule.

Walking

One of the most effective yet underestimated exercises is walking. Some experts suggest that walking can be a great exercise, maybe even better than running (Steinhilber, 2020). I understand that time to walk can be scarce, especially when your schedule is quite tight. At your workplace, you could choose to walk the steps rather than using the elevator to the next floor of the building! It is easy to underestimate the efficacy of walking as an exercise when you compare it with other exercises like cycling, running, and other cardio exercises but wait until you hear its proven benefits:

- **Your heart health is improved:** Researchers reported that walking plays a crucial role in reducing the risk of cardiovascular diseases in males and females, both the young and the old (Murtagh, 2010). The scientists that did this study even recommended that clinicians should prescribe walking to their patients so that they can meet physical activity benchmarks. In yet another study, it was shown that participants who walked for at least 40 minutes in a week at a moderate or fast pace had a reduced risk of heart failure by about 25% (Napoli, 2018).
- **Improved cholesterol ratios:** You are healthier when the level of High Density Lipoproteins (HDL) is higher than that of Low Density Lipoproteins (LDL). HDLs help to remove excess cholesterol from your body, therefore reducing the possibility of cholesterol-

clogged arteries. LDLs act in the reverse and promote the accumulation of cholesterol in the arteries, and this increases the risk of heart failure. The good news is that walking reduces the amounts of LDLs, while increasing the HDLs. Results from a study showed that walking can reduce the concentration of LDLs in the blood by 4% (Wang & Xu, 2017).

- **Reduced risk of type 2 diabetes:** By just walking for at least 30 minutes per day, participants in a study experienced a 50% decrease in the risk of type 2 diabetes (Hamasaki, 2016). Type 2 diabetes is a condition where the body fails to engage insulin in aiding cells to take up glucose. This causes blood sugar levels to rise.

Turn Your House Chores Into Exercises

Do you feel like you have too much on your plate, and you can't leave your hose chores for some form of exercise? I got you covered with this idea of creating exercise out of the house chores that you possibly do every day. This could be anything from dusting off your ceiling to washing your car. It's all in the head. The stretching that you might possibly do while leaving your house chore unattended can still be done while you attend to them. As you reach out with your broom, you are stretching some muscles and engaging your body. The energy that you put in as you vacuum your floors—that can be a lot of exercise if you let it.

Have you ever tried some wall sits while you neatly fold your clothes? How about some squats? You will be surprised at how much you will be sweating by the time you finish your chores, much more than you have ever done before. You will benefit more from these exercises when you do them on a regular basis.

Make Classic Squats Part of Your Bathing Routine

You are already up and standing, so instead of just rushing to the bathroom for your bath, how about coupling that with some squats? You can do this regularly until the two become inseparable for you. If you are not sure about how to do the classic squat, the instructions that I have listed below could be just for you:

1. Stand with your feet apart. The distance between your feet should be about shoulder width. Your toes should be facing toward the front.
2. Lower your butt by gradually bending your knees. Do this until you feel a burning sensation in your thighs. Ensure that knees do not surpass your toe-tips.
3. Maintain this position for two seconds before you stand up.
4. Repeat steps (1) to (3) no less than 10 times.

End the Day With Some Wall Push-Ups

Wrapping up a busy day with some wall push-ups can be great. If this moment overlaps into your fasting window of intermittent fasting, that would be even more ideal. Follow the below steps for some wall push-ups:

1. Make sure your hands are clean to avoid messing your walls.
2. Stand while facing the wall, at a distance of about 15 inches. The distance could be slightly less or more, depending on your stature.
3. Place your hands on the wall, at a height that is in line with your shoulders.
4. Bend your elbows, either upward or downwards whichever way is best for you. The aim is to bring your chest closer to the wall, while your feet remain in their previous position.
5. By stretching your arms, push yourself back to your upright standing position.
6. Repeat steps (1) to (5) at least 10 times.

Circuit Exercises

Sometimes, it is difficult to identify just one exercise that you want to engage in on a regular basis. Circuit exercises can be a good option in that case. In circuit exercises, you select a few exercises that you do one after the other in sort of a "cycle." For example, you may begin with a set of push-ups, skip with a skipping rope for four minutes, do a set of resistance band curls, and complete the circuit with shadow boxing for two minutes. You can repeat the circuit as many times as you prefer.

Circuit exercise is good, especially when you are working with limited time. You decide for yourself which exercises you want to include in a particular circuit and how long you want each exercise to take. Besides, focusing on one exercise for a long time can be disengaging sometimes. Constant switches between exercises can be a great way to spice up your workouts.

Chapter 7: How to Succeed in LCIF and Stay Healthy

Intermittent fasting has its best results when it's done consistently over a long period of time. In fact, it should become more like a habit and lifestyle so that you reap the lifelong benefits of the practice. However, just like any other endeavor that has benefits, intermittent fasting has its own ups and downs. You may wake up feeling helplessly hungry when you are supposed to be fasting. You can get sick and get medications that require you to eat first. Not to mention naysayers who will tell you that you are wasting your time. The list is endless but not long enough to stop you from making intermittent fasting your lifestyle. This is the reason why you need to set up strategies that keep you focused and committed to doing intermittent fasting, no matter what comes your way. This section is dedicated to helping you to find more reasons for doing intermittent fasting. After all, the benefits outweigh the negatives.

Before we delve into more tips on how to keep going with LCIF, I would like to briefly discuss one tip that can be of great help. Having some cheat days may help you not to feel cocooned by the LCIF procedures.

You Can Have Some Cheat Days

A cheat day is a day when you consciously sway from your normal and ideal eating patterns. In other words, you will be breaking your own adopted rules and principles that are the foundations of your diet and eating patterns. Mind you, it's only for a day, after which you go back to your normal eating routines.

Cheating days in intermittent fasting are less focused on what you are going to eat, but more on when you are going to eat. You intentionally break the rules that stipulate when you are going to eat. Simply said, you eat during the time when you are supposed to be fasting. You can do this by extending the feasting period into your fasting window or by completely skipping the whole fasting window.

What you eat on a cheat day only becomes important if the reason for your fasting is, say, to lower your blood glucose levels. In this case, then eating foods such as donuts, which contain high amounts of sugars, becomes "cheating" on your normal eating patterns (Conway, 2020).

It is completely fine for you to have cheat days. However, before you set it up, you should give yourself honest answers to the following questions:

- Why are you doing intermittent fasting? If it is for you to manage certain health conditions, then cheating by eating food that is harmful to you might not be such a great decision.
- Are you hungry at the time that you are "cheating"?
- Did you plan the cheat day or maybe you just wanted to honor an invitation from a friend? If the cheating

was not planned, you can compensate for the eating hours by starting your next fast a bit earlier.

My Testimony

I normally do the 14-hour fasting type. When I started practising intermittent fasting, I did my cheat days on weekends. As time passed by, I eventually didn't have to do cheat days anymore, most probably because I progressively became used to my fasting period. I am 53 years old, and somehow, I manage to maintain my desired weight. It's amazing because in 2019, when I started fasting intermittently, I wouldn't do it daily, but when I started seeing that it worked, I became more focused and committed to it, and it ultimately became a habit!

More Tips

Here are more tips that help you to maintain your grip on practising LCIF:

1. **Choose the appropriate fasting type:** The danger that lies in choosing a fasting routine that does not suit you is that you can easily give up when the going gets tough. Choose the fasting hours that you can manage and sustain. You might also need to consider the time

of the day when your fasting window will begin and end. It is more difficult to endure fasting in the afternoons in extremely hot climates or seasons. In such climates, avoiding fasting windows that include afternoons can be daunting.

2. **Avoid storing foods that you might binge on:** Keeping foods that you can easily binge on is not a good idea. It is more probable that when you conclude your fasting, you will be feeling hungry, and binging is one of the things that you will want to avoid at all costs. It counters your efforts of fasting by causing surges in blood sugar levels in the body. At the end of the day, you might end up feeling more hungry than before.

3. **Strategize on how to go through hunger peaks:** There are times when you will feel extremely hungry while in the middle of a fast. The urge to give up and eat will be so overwhelming, but you still have to keep on. This is why you should come up with strategies that help you to go through this tempting moment. You can keep yourself busy with something to shift your focus from hunger. Alternatively, you can learn and adopt the art of ignoring the hunger until it subsides on its own. This usually has the best results if you master it well.

4. **Avoid alcohol:** Alcohol is not your best companion when it comes to intermittent fasting. There are many reasons for this. Alcohol makes you feel hungrier, it disturbs metabolism, and prevents loss of fat, in addition to sapping your energy.

5. **Be part of a support community:** Having people that encourage you on your fasting endeavor is a good

step. These could be people that you choose to share your successes, challenges, and failures with. They could be friends, family, or colleagues. It might be best to be part of a group of people who are also doing LCIF. Such people understand you better, and their encouragement sounds more realistic.

6. **Keep yourself hydrated:** Drinking water, tea, or coffee is allowed when you are fasting. These liquids will help to keep you hydrated. You are also less likely to feel hungry when there are some liquids in your stomach. The liquids stretch your intestines a bit, making you feel fuller. This way, you will be better able to keep going.

7. **Eat to satiation:** When you are done with a day's fasting, eat as much as you like, but only up to satiation. Do not keep eating because this will only make LCIF more difficult to sustain. The same applies to your last meals before your next fasting window. Most people are tempted to eat more in preparation for fasting. You cannot cover up for the food that you will miss when you fast. If you eat more food to reduce the chances of feeling hungry, you are worsening the situation. You are more likely to feel hungrier than you would after normal eating.

8. **Take note of how you feel:** It is important to always be attentive to your body. When you feel good as a result of your fasting, take note of it; it is good-enough motivation to keep you focused on LCIF. When you notice signs such as dizziness, headache, fatigue, anxiety, and lack of focus, do not take them lightly. They might be alerting you that something is

wrong in your body, and not attending to these signs and symptoms might aggravate situations. I recommend that you break your fast immediately when you experience these and other uncomfortable signs.

9. **Focus on protein and fiber-rich foods:** When you eat, make it a habit to focus on foods that are rich in fiber and proteins. Such foods will help you to feel fuller for longer. That implies that you won't be overwhelmed by the urge to eat while you are fasting. Generally, protein and fiber-rich foods are low in calories. Eating more carbohydrates is the last thing that you want to do. Carbohydrates are quick sources of energy to the body, and therefore they are quickly used up. As a result, you will feel hungry more frequently. This makes fasting difficult, while making you eat more than is necessary during your feasting window.

10. **Exercise appropriately:** Exercise is good, but it can be dangerous when it is done inappropriately. When you are not fasting, it is fine to do any exercise, even the strenuous ones. Go ahead and lift those heavy weights and run marathons, as long as it's not during the fasting window. When you are fasting, stick to light exercises like walking, stretching, and light yoga. Exercise requires energy, which your body does not have during exercise. Remember, your body processes are actually depending on your fatty reserves.

Chapter 8: 10 Yummy Recipes to Start Your Journey

Garlic Chicken Thighs Dipped in Mushroom Sauce

Lick your fingers with this yummy recipe. Garlic-flavored chicken thighs are something that you won't regret trying, especially when they are dipped in mushroom sauce (Cherrier, 2021). Give this a try and in **20 minutes'** time, your meal will be ready for you to enjoy with your loved ones.

Ingredients

- Sun-dried and oiled tomatoes (5 ounces)
- Skinless and deboned chicken thighs (5)
- Finely sliced garlic (5 cloves)
- Chicken broth (⅓ cup)
- Sliced mushrooms (3 cups)
- Butter (2 tablespoons)
- Salt (added to taste)
- Small yellow onion cut into medium dice (1 bulb)
- Grated Parmesan (½ cup)
- Pepper (added to taste)
- Chopped, fresh parsley (1 tablespoon)
- Heavy whipping cream (1 ¾ cup)

Instructions

1. ***Prepare the chicken thighs:*** Switch your stove to a medium-to-high heat range while you pour the cooking oil into a large frying pan. Allow it to heat. Use salt and pepper to completely season the chicken thighs. Add the chicken into the frying pan with the heated oil for five minutes, before you turn it over to cook the other side. Take the chicken thighs out of the skillet when they are cooked through (in about 10 minutes' time).

2. ***Prepare the mushrooms:*** Add the butter to the same pan and with the same heat range, until it melts. Put the sliced mushrooms into the pan and gently stir them until they attain a golden-brown color on all sides.

3. ***Add the flavors:*** Add garlic to the well-cooked mushrooms and let them stand for approximately a minute, to allow for the garlic fragrance to come out. Add the diced yellow onions and fry them until they are semitransparent. Put the sun-dried tomatoes into the pan and fry until their flavors also come out. This might take about two minutes. Pour the chicken broth into the skillet and give it time to reduce down.

4. ***Prepare the mushroom sauce:*** Reduce your cooking heat to low and allow the stove to adjust, prior to adding the heavy whipping cream. Leave the pan contents to simmer, while you stir from time to time. As in step (1), use salt and pepper to season the sauce to your preferable taste. Add the Parmesan cheese while the creamy mushroom sauce simmers so that it melts. This might take two minutes.

5. ***Make the creamy garlic chicken thighs in mushroom sauce:*** Get the already-cooked chicken thighs that you set aside in (1) above and add them back into the pan. Sprinkle the parsley onto the chicken before adding the sauce over each piece, using the cooking spoon.

6. ***Serving suggestion:*** You can serve the yummy garlic chicken thighs in mushroom sauce over steamed vegetables or rice.

Cucumber Submarine Sandwich With Turkey

Are you craving a sub sandwich? This cucumber sub sandwich will fulfill your cravings, while you cut down on the carbohydrates that usually come with sub sandwiches (Webster, 2017). It's like hitting two birds with one stone.

Ingredients

- Peeled cucumber (1 large)
- Swiss cheese (½ ounce)
- Thin slices of tomatoes (3)
- Mayonnaise (2 teaspoons)
- Thin slice of white onion (1)
- Yellow mustard (2 teaspoons)
- Sliced turkey breasts (2 ounces)
- Ground pepper

1. **Prepare the cucumber:** Use a knife to cut the cucumber in half in a lengthwise direction. Remove all the seeds from the inside of the cucumber halves so that they become hollowed. Place the cucumber pieces down on a clean surface, such that the cut sides face up.

2. **Make your sub sandwich:** Smoothly spread mayonnaise and yellow mustard on the inside of the cucumber halves. On one half of the cucumber, layer the turkey first, followed by the Swiss cheese. Neatly place the three tomato slices on top of the cheese. Add the onions in the gaps that are left by the tomatoes. Sprinkle the ground pepper for seasoning. Close your sandwich by placing the other half of the cucumber on top, with the cut side facing downwards, toward the tomatoes.

3. **Serving suggestion**: There is your cucumber submarine sandwich with turkey. Cut it into halves and enjoy!

Cajun-Spiced Shrimp Sausage in Foil

Enjoy your shrimp, summer vegetables, sausages, and Cajun spices, all wrapped in one piece of aluminum foil. With an approximate cooking time of *15 minutes*, you are assured of your healthy, low-carbohydrate meal in less than 30 minutes (Cherrier, 2020).

Ingredients

- Sliced, smoked pork sausage (14 ounces)
- Peeled and deveined shrimp (1 pound)
- Butter (2 tablespoons)
- Sliced zucchini (1 medium sized)
- Cajun seasoning (2 tablespoons)
- Salt and pepper (½ teaspoon)
- Vegetable stock (2 tablespoons)
- Minced garlic (3 cloves)
- Trimmed asparagus, chopped into chunks
- Diced red bell paper (1)

Instructions

1. ***Prepare to start:*** Begin by preheating the oven to 425□F. While the oven adjusts to the set temperature, use scissors to prepare two aluminum foil pieces that are 14-by-12 inches in size. Place them on a separate position on the countertop.

2. ***Get the sausage and shrimp ready:*** Divide the sausage and shrimp that you have into two equal parts and share them between the two aluminum foil pieces that you spread on the countertop. Make sure they are at the center of the foil. Place the asparagus and bell pepper on the side of the shrimps and sausages. Sprinkle generous amounts of the Cajun seasoning on all the contents on the foil.

3. ***Add some flavors:*** Spread the minced garlic on all the foil piece contents. Get the butter, divide it into two, and lay it over the shrimp and vegetables on each of the foil pieces.
4. ***It's time to bake:*** Add the vegetable stock, one tablespoon in each foil packet. Carefully wrap the foil packets and be sure to keep them slightly loose to allow for free circulation of heat. Transfer both foil packets to the baking tray and put them in the oven. Make sure the sealed sides of the foil packets are facing upwards. In about 15 minutes, the shrimps, sausages, and veggies are well cooked.
5. ***Serving suggestion:*** Garnish the baked shrimp, sausages, and veggies with one slice of lemon and fresh parsley.

First-Class Egg and Bacon

Try this easy to make and seemingly simple meal, and you will find no reason not to try it again. It is simple but satisfying (Aobadia, 2021).

Ingredients

- Large eggs (8)
- Diced cherry tomatoes (half a handful)
- Sliced bacon (9 ounces or 255 grams)
- Fresh thyme

Instructions

1. ***Prepare the bacon:*** Put the pan over medium to high heat. Add the bacon and fry it until it is crispy. Take it out and put it aside on a plate. Do not remove the bacon fat from the pan.
2. ***Prepare the eggs:*** Crack your eggs into a measuring cup and carefully add them to the pan with the bacon oil, to avoid spilling. Cook your eggs using the "sunny side up" method. Do not flip your egg. Instead, cover the pan with a lid to ensure that the top is fully cooked as well.
3. ***Flavors and seasoning:*** Add the cut cherry tomatoes into the frying pan with the eggs. Fry them together with the eggs. Add the fresh thyme for its flavor before you add salt and pepper, to your taste.
4. ***Serving suggestion:*** Eat this as a light meal.

Cabbage and Chicken in Egg Roll Bowls

Not only is this egg roll bowl with cabbage and chicken recipe easy to follow, it is also very nourishing (Cherrier, 2020). This low-carb and gluten-free meal takes only **10 minutes** to prepare, and in no time, the food will be on your table.

Ingredients

- Ground turkey (1 pound)
- Crushed red pepper (1 teaspoon)

- Garlic powder (1 tablespoon)
- Chicken broth (½ cup)
- Sliced green onions (2 bulbs)
- Soy sauce (1 tablespoon)
- Minced onion (1 medium sized)
- Vegetable oil (2 tablespoons)
- Ginger powder (1 tablespoon)
- Preshredded coleslaw mix (1 bag)
- Salt and pepper (½ teaspoon of each)
- Hot sauce of your choice (1 tablespoon)
- Chopped chives

Cooking Method

1. ***Prepare the turkey meat:*** Add the vegetable oil in a pan and heat it at medium to high temperature. Add the turkey meat into the pan and cook until it becomes brownish. Add the onion (not the green onions) to the pan and continue cooking until the onions are slightly brown in color.

2. ***Flavor it up:*** Get the ginger, garlic powder, and all peppers and add them to the meat and onions in the pan. Stir well to mix the pan contents. Before adding the coleslaw mix and the green onion, add the chicken broth first.

3. ***Add in the vegetable:*** Add the cabbage and cook it to tenderness. Remember to stir from time to time.

4. ***Saucing:*** It's time to add the sauces, that is, soy sauce and that other hot sauce of your choice. Add salt and pepper to your desired taste and continue stirring.

5. ***Serving suggestion:*** Use chopped chives for garnishing and add your prepared food into bowls. You can serve it as it is or over cauliflower rice.

Avocados Stuffed With Salmon

Salmon is a great source of omega-3 fatty acids, which you definitely need in your body. These avocados that are stuffed with salmon are a good choice if you are not planning on turning your stove on to cook (Gellmann, 2019). Eat healthy with this yummy and easy-to-make recipe.

Ingredients

- Fresh, chopped parsley (2 tablespoons)
- Mayonnaise (2 tablespoons)
- Lime juice (1 tablespoon)
- Dijon mustard (1 teaspoon)
- Diced celery (½ cup)
- Plain Greek yogurt (½ cup)
- Salt and ground pepper (⅛ teaspoon of each)
- Chopped chives
- Avocados (2 each)
- Drained, flaked, deboned salmon, with removed skin (2 cans or 5 ounces)

Instructions

1. ***Prepare the avocados:*** With a knife, cut the avocados in the lengthwise direction, to make two halves. Fill a tablespoon with the flesh from one half of the avocados and transfer it into a small bowl. Do the same for the other halves. Use a fork to mash all the avocado flesh in the small bowl.

2. ***Prepare the other ingredients:*** Get a medium-sized bowl and add mayonnaise, celery, yogurt, lime juice, mustard, parsley, pepper, and salt. Mix well before you add the salmon. Mix again after adding the salmon.

3. ***Prepare the complete filling:*** Transfer the mashed avocados into the mixture of salmon and other ingredients in the medium-sized bowl. Thoroughly mix. What you have after mixing is your salmon filling.

4. ***Stuff the avocados:*** Use the salmon filling to stuff the avocado halves. Do this by adding a half-cup measure of the salmon filling into each of the avocado halves. Use chives to garnish. Your salmon-stuffed avocado is ready!

Cauliflower Rice Muffins

These gluten-free muffins are made up of cauliflower rice, instead of flour (Meyer, 2018). Enjoy the unique appearance, flavors, and experience of eating a cauliflower rice muffin.

Ingredients

- Cauliflower florets (5 cups or 1 pound)
- Lightly beaten egg (1 large)
- Salt (⅛ teaspoon)
- Shredded Cheddar cheese (1 cup)

Instructions

1. ***Get prepared:*** While you preheat the oven to 425□F, start lining the baking sheet that you are going to use with baking paper.

2. ***Prepare the cauliflower rice:*** Wash your cauliflower clean, before you place it in a food processor for grating. Remove the finely grated cauliflower from the food processor and place it in a microwave-safe bowl. Microwave on high for not more than three minutes, ensuring that the bowl with the cauliflower is slightly covered. Take the bowl out and allow it to cool down. Spread a clean kitchen cloth on your working space and transfer the cauliflower to it. Completely cover the cauliflower with the kitchen cloth and wring until the cauliflower is as dry as possible. Meanwhile, add the egg, Cheddar cheese, and salt into the bowl. Add the cauliflower into the same bowl and mix thoroughly.

3. ***Ready to bake?:*** Take a three-inch biscuit cutter and place it on the baking sheet that you prepared. Add about a quarter cup of the batter to the biscuit cutter and slightly pat the batter down in the mold. Use the remaining batter to prepare seven more muffins in the same way that you prepared the first one. There should be a space of one inch between each of your cauliflower muffins. Place the baking sheet into the preheated oven and bake until the edges of the muffins are brownish and crispy. This should take approximately 25 minutes.

4. ***Serving suggestion:*** You can serve the yummy cauliflower muffins with sweet jam or any other topping of your choice.

Avocado and Shrimp Salad

You want to have shrimp or an avocado? How about making this avocado shrimp salad and enjoying both of them at once? Besides being a healthy, low-carbohydrate meal, your taste buds will surely appreciate it. You can prepare this meal in less than 5 minutes (Cherrier, 2020).

Ingredients

- Raw, peeled, and deveined shrimp (8 ounces or 250 grams)
- Lime juice (1 tablespoon)
- Minced red onion (½ bulb)
- Pepper and salt (add to taste)
- Diced avocado (1 large)
- Chopped parsley
- Premelted salted butter (2 tablespoons)
- Olive oil (1 tablespoon)
- Diced cherry tomatoes (1 handful)

Instructions

1. ***Prepare the shrimp:*** Add the shrimp to the premelted butter and toss it until it is completely coated with the butter.

2. ***Cook the shrimp:*** Heat the frying pan over a medium to high heat prior to adding the shrimp. Sear the shrimp until you begin to notice some pink edges. This should be in a minute's time. Flip the shrimp over to the other side. Allow it cook until the whole shrimp is well cooked. Ideally, this should be in less than a minute's time. Remove the shrimp from the pan and place it on a shallow plate so that it cools.

3. ***Prepare the other ingredients:*** Add the red onion, parsley, tomatoes, and avocado into a mixing bowl. After adding the olive oil and the lime juice respectively, toss the mixing bowl so that its contents are well mixed.

4. ***Make the salad:*** Add the cooked and cooled shrimp into the mixing bowl with the other ingredients. Gently mix well. Add the salt and pepper to the salad, to taste.

5. ***Serving suggestion:*** You can consider serving the avocado shrimp salad over toasted bread.

Parmesan Cauliflower Rice

Parmesan cauliflower rice is a good base for your meals when you are on a low-carbohydrate diet (Cherrier, 2021). Replace the high -carbohydrate rice recipes with low-carbohydrate cauliflower rice ones. In not more than 20 minutes, food will be served.

Ingredients

- Grated cauliflower (1 head)
- Finely grated, fresh Parmesan (2 ounces)
- Unsalted butter (2 tablespoons)
- Juice from a half lemon
- Minced garlic (2 cloves)
- Chopped fresh parsley
- Chopped white onion (½ of a bulb)
- Red chili pepper flakes (1 teaspoon)
- Vegetable stock (2 tablespoons)

Cooking Method

1. ***Prepare the butter, garlic, and onion:*** Place your pan over medium to high heat. Melt 2 tablespoons of butter in the pan, prior to adding onions and garlic. Fry these for not more than a minute to ensure that they are not burnt.
2. ***Prepare the cauliflower:*** Add the cauliflower rice into the same pan. Mix everything well by regular stirring until all the pan contents are coated in butter. This might take about a minute.
3. ***Add the flavors:*** Add half the parsley, together with the vegetable stock into the pan. After a minute of cooking, add parmesan cheese and the juice that you squeezed from the half lemon. Adjust the seasoning as you deem appropriate. Stir in the remaining parsley.

4. **Serving suggestion:** Consider serving your parmesan cauliflower rice with red chili pepper flakes and coarsely ground black pepper.

Supergreen Yummy Smoothie

Instead of just having your low-carb meals through eating, you can drink them. Sounds interesting, doesn't it? Learn how to prepare a yummy supergreen smoothie within 10 minutes.

Ingredients

- Young spinach leaves (1 handful)
- Juiced lime (1)
- Peeled and chunked cucumber (¼)
- Juiced kiwi fruit (1 large)
- Peeled and chunked avocado (¼ avocado)

Cooking Method

1. *Prepare your smoothie in one step:* Place the avocado, cucumber, spinach, as well as the lime and kiwi fruit juices in a blender. Whizz them until they are smooth.
2. *Serving suggestion:* You can drink the smoothie as it is, or you can add a little water to dilute.

Conclusion

Just by a single search on the internet, thousands of diets will pop up, each with its own promises for healthy benefits, weight loss, and sustainability. The experience that we have had with most of these diets makes us skeptical as to what really works. Most of the diets focus on what should be eaten, and in most cases, what should not be eaten. With the strict stipulation of what should and should not be eaten, your choices do not matter much. You simply have to follow the instructions to the T, which is often difficult, considering that the new diet might be completely different to your previous diet.

Intermittent fasting is not a diet; it is a lifestyle. In this case, the focus is not on what should or should not be eaten, but on when to eat. That said, intermittent fasting is done by scheduling eating and fasting periods in an alternating manner such that a feasting window if followed by a fasting window. There are different types of intermittent fasting that exist, and you have the leeway to choose what suits your preferences. Some prefer to fast on selected days of a week. Some prefer to alternate days of fasting and those of feasting. Most prefer to select hours of fasting and feasting in a single day. In all cases, the length of the fasting period differs. In intermittent fasting, it is the length of the fasting window that counts, not that of the feasting window. This is because the benefits of the practice depend on your fasting as opposed to eating patterns.

Intermittent fasting is coupled with various benefits. For those who want to lose and then maintain their desired weight, intermittent fasting could be your answer. When your body goes without food for 10 hours or more, it will have to use up the glycogen reserves in the liver. For that reason, the body will turn to its fat reserves for energy. The breakdown of fats to produce energy reduces accumulation of fats in the body. This equally impacts weight loss.

The unavailability of food in the stomach during fasting improves the efficiency of bodily processes. When the gut is full of food, more focus and energy is channeled toward processes such as digestion and absorption, and related processes. When there is no food in the body, there is more energy to spare, which can be directed toward improving the efficiency of other processes in the body. This way, fasting enhances metabolism.

Fasting is also associated with rejuvenating the body, as well as delaying aging in natural ways. Just in the same way that you feel energized and more focused after a deep sleep, fasting has more or less the same effects on the body. When there is food and excess energy in the body, there are a lot of activities that will be going on in the body. Enzymes, neurons, neurotransmitters, and hormones have more work to do. More waste is released by cellular processes, and excretory processes are triggered. Simply said, the body's components are more engaged when you are not fasting. When you are fasting, the body is in a more relaxed state, which is rejuvenating.

LCIF recommends that you eat low-carbohydrate foods during your feasting window. This means cutting down on highly starchy foods like rice and turning to foods like vegetables, fruits, and lean meats which have low carbohydrate content. It is recommended that you eat more proteins, fibers, and healthy fats. This does not, however, mean that you cannot give yourself some treats once in a while You can, but you should be able to go back to your eating patterns soon after that.

Intermittent fasting can be demanding, especially when you are not used to it. However, there are many strategies that you can employ to cruise through the ups and down that are associated with fasting intermittently. Some of these are highlighted in this book. This book ends with a list of detailed, yummy low-carbohydrate recipes that are easy and can be prepared in less time. Check them out and enjoy yourself, together with your family, colleagues, and friends!

References

14 easy (and sneaky) ways to exercise for busy people. (2019, April 17). The Budding Optimist. https://buddingoptimist.com/ways-to-exercise/

Aging changes in body shape: MedlinePlus Medical Encyclopedia. (n.d.). Medlineplus.gov. Retrieved February 19, 2021, from https://medlineplus.gov/ency/article/003998.htm

Alirezaei, M., Kemball, C. C., Flynn, C. T., Wood, M. R., Whitton, J. L., & Kiosses, W. B. (2010). Short-term fasting induces profound neuronal autophagy. Autophagy, 6(6), 702–710. https://doi.org/10.4161/auto.6.6.12376

Aly, S. M. (2014). Role of intermittent fasting on improving health and reducing diseases. International Journal of Health Sciences, 8(3), V–VI. https://www.ncbi.nlm.nih.gov/pmc/articles/PMC42 57368/

Aobadia, A. (2021, February 10). Keto bacon and eggs — Classic breakfast recipe. Diet Doctor. https://www.dietdoctor.com/recipes/classic-bacon-and-eggs

Arumugam, T. V., Phillips, T. M., Cheng, A., Morrell, C. H., Mattson, M. P., & Wan, R. (2010). Age and energy intake interact to modify cell stress pathways and stroke outcome. Annals of Neurology, 67(1), 41–52. https://doi.org/10.1002/ana.21798

Bacharach, E. (2019, November 18). *A fasting diet shouldn't turn you into a hangry betch—Here's how to do it right.* Women's Health. https://www.womenshealthmag.com/weight-loss/a29602869/fasting-tips/

Brazier, Y. (2020, January 18). *How much should I weigh for my height and age? BMI calculator.* www.medicalnewstoday.com. https://www.medicalnewstoday.com/articles/32344 6

Bumgardner, W. (2016, February 20). *Ideal weight by height calculator chart.* Verywell Fit. https://www.verywellfit.com/ideal-weight-calculator-chart-3878254

Cherrier, C. (2020, December 1). *Cajun sausage shrimp vegetable foil packs recipe – Shrimp and sausage foil packets recipe.* www.eatwell101.com. https://www.eatwell101.com/cajun-shrimp-sausage-foil-packs-recipe

Cherrier, C. (2020, January 2). *Easy shrimp avocado salad with tomatoes.* Eatwell101. https://www.eatwell101.com/shrimp-avocado-salad-recipe

Cherrier, C. (2020, August 6). *Egg roll bowls recipe with chicken and cabbage —* www.eatwell101.com. https://www.eatwell101.com/egg-roll-bowls-recipe

Cherrier, C. (2021, March 11). *Garlic chicken thighs recipe in creamy mushroom sauce – Chicken thighs recipe.* www.eatwell101.com. https://www.eatwell101.com/creamy-chicken-thighs-recipe

Cherrier, C. (2021, January 28). *Parmesan cauliflower rice skillet recipe – Cauliflower rice recipes.* www.eatwell101.com. https://www.eatwell101.com/parmesan-cauliflower-rice-skillet

Clear, J. (2012, December 10). *The beginner's guide to intermittent fasting.* James Clear. https://jamesclear.com/the-beginners-guide-to-intermittent-fasting

Cleveland Clinic. (n.d.). *Healthy fat intake.* Cleveland Clinic. https://my.clevelandclinic.org/health/articles/11208-fat-what-you-need-to-know

Collier, R. (2013). Intermittent fasting: The science of going without. *Canadian Medical Association Journal, 185*(9), E363–E364. https://doi.org/10.1503/cmaj.109-4451

Conway, S.-M. (2020, March 26). *Having a cheat day while intermittent fasting.* Simple.life blog. https://simple.life/blog/cheat-day-during-intermittent-fasting/

Correll, C. U., Lencz, T., & Malhotra, A. K. (2011). Antipsychotic drugs and obesity. *Trends in Molecular Medicine, 17*(2), 97–107. https://doi.org/10.1016/j.molmed.2010.10.010

Debara, D. (2019, January 16). *5 rules to weighing yourself — and when to ditch the scale.* Healthline. https://www.healthline.com/health/fitness-exercises/weigh-yourself-guidelines

Drayer, L. (2018, March 23). *How to succeed at intermittent fasting.* CNN.

https://edition.cnn.com/2018/03/23/health/intermittent-fasting-food-drayer/index.html

Eenfeldt, A. (2021). *Carbs on low carb: How low carb is low carb?* Diet Doctor. https://www.dietdoctor.com/low-carb/how-low-carb-is-low-carb

Faris, M. A.-I. E., Kacimi, S., Al-Kurd, R. A., Fararjeh, M. A., Bustanji, Y. K., Mohammad, M. K., and Salem, M. L. (2012). Intermittent fasting during Ramadan attenuates proinflammatory cytokines and immune cells in healthy subjects. *Nutrition Research, 32*(12), 947–955. https://doi.org/10.1016/j.nutres.2012.06.021

Fletcher, M. (2010, September 30). *How is excess glucose stored?* Livestron.com. https://www.livestrong.com/article/264767-how-is-excess-glucose-stored/

Frey, M. (2016). *Bioelectrical impedance analysis (BIA).* Verywell Fit. https://www.verywellfit.com/bioelectrical-impedance-analysis-bia-3495551

Ganesan, K., Habboush, Y., & Sultan, S. (2018). Intermittent fasting: The Choice for a Healthier Lifestyle. *Cureus, 10*(7). https://doi.org/10.7759/cureus.2947

Gellmann, A. (2019). *Salmon-stuffed avocados.* EatingWell. https://www.eatingwell.com/recipe/270549/salmon-stuffed-avocados/

Gunnars, K. (2020, September 25). *How intermittent fasting can help you lose weight.* Healthline. https://www.healthline.com/nutrition/intermittent-fasting-and-weight-loss

Gunners, K. (2020, October 2). *Protein intake — How much protein should you eat per day?* Healthline. https://www.healthline.com/nutrition/how-much-protein-per-day

Hamasaki, H. (2016). Daily physical activity and type 2 diabetes: A review. *World Journal of Diabetes, 7*(12), 243. https://doi.org/10.4239/wjd.v7.i12.243

Harvard Health Publishing. (2019, June 24). *Why people become overweight.* Harvard Health. https://www.health.harvard.edu/staying-healthy/why-people-become-overweight

Hatori, M., Vollmers, C., Zarrinpar, A., DiTacchio, L., Bushong, Eric A., Gill, S., Leblanc, M., Chaix, A., Joens, M., Fitzpatrick, James A. J., Ellisman, Mark H., & Panda, S. (2012). Time-restricted feeding without reducing caloric intake prevents Metabolic Diseases in Mice Fed a High-Fat Diet. *Cell Metabolism, 15*(6), 848–860. https://doi.org/10.1016/j.cmet.2012.04.019

Hazell, A. (2019). *BMI formula - How to use the BMI formula.* Thecalculatorsite.com. https://www.thecalculatorsite.com/articles/health/bmi-formula-for-bmi-calculations.php

Heilbronn, L. K., Civitarese, A. E., Bogacka, I., Smith, S. R., Hulver, M., & Ravussin, E. (2005). Glucose tolerance and skeletal muscle gene expression in response to alternate day fasting. *Obesity Research, 13*(3), 574–581. https://doi.org/10.1038/oby.2005.61

Heilbronn, L. K., Smith, S. R., Martin, C. K., Anton, S. D., & Ravussin, E. (2005). Alternate-day fasting in nonobese subjects: effects on body weight, body composition, and energy metabolism. *The American Journal of Clinical Nutrition*, *81*(1), 69–73. https://doi.org/10.1093/ajcn/81.1.69

Ho, K. Y., Veldhuis, J. D., Johnson, M. L., Furlanetto, R., Evans, W. S., Alberti, K. G., & Thorner, M. O. (1988). Fasting enhances growth hormone secretion and amplifies the complex rhythms of growth hormone secretion in man. *Journal of Clinical Investigation*, *81*(4), 968–975. https://doi.org/10.1172/jci113450

How the body decreases blood glucose concentrations after eating. (n.d.). FutureLearn. https://www.futurelearn.com/info/courses/understanding-insulin/0/steps/22455

Jarreau, P. B. (2018, May 9). *Your questions about intermittent fasting, answered (Part 1).* Medium. https://medium.com/lifeomic/your-questions-about-intermittent-fasting-answered-part-1-7b770594690b

Johnson, J. B., Summer, W., Cutler, R. G., Martin, B., Hyun, D.-H., Dixit, V. D., Pearson, M., Nassar, M., Tellejohan, R., Maudsley, S., Carlson, O., John, S., Laub, D. R., & Mattson, M. P. (2007). Alternate day calorie restriction improves clinical findings and reduces markers of oxidative stress and inflammation in overweight adults with moderate asthma. *Free Radical Biology and Medicine*, *42*(5), 665–674. https://doi.org/10.1016/j.freeradbiomed.2006.12.005

Kamb, S. (2019, July 29). *Intermittent fasting for beginners: Should you skip breakfast?* Nerd Fitness. https://www.nerdfitness.com/blog/a-beginners-guide-to-intermittent-fasting/

Kretzschmer, W. (2020, February 21). *Intermittent fasting 101: Fast. Feast. Repeat.* www.onemedical.com. https://www.onemedical.com/blog/eat-well/intermittent-fasting

Kubala, J. (2019, April 23). *6 ways added sugar is fattening.* Healthline. https://www.healthline.com/nutrition/does-sugar-make-you-fat

Lawler, M. (2020, March 17). *12 burning questions about intermittent fasting, answered.* EverydayHealth.com. https://www.everydayhealth.com/diet-nutrition/burning-questions-about-intermittent-fasting-answered/

Lee, J., Duan, W., Long, J. M., Ingram, D. K., & Mattson, M. P. (2000). Dietary restriction increases the number of newly generated neural cells, and induces BDNF expression, in the dentate gyrus of Rats. *Journal of Molecular Neuroscience, 15*(2), 99–108. https://doi.org/10.1385/jmn:15:2:99

Leonard, J. (2020, April 16). *7 ways to do intermittent fasting: Best methods and quick tips.* www.medicalnewstoday.com. https://www.medicalnewstoday.com/articles/322293

Li, L., Wang, Z., & Zuo, Z. (2013). Chronic intermittent fasting improves cognitive functions and brain structures in mice. *PloS One, 8*(6), e66069. https://doi.org/10.1371/journal.pone.0066069

Loucks, A. B., & Thuma, J. R. (2003). Luteinizing hormone pulsatility is disrupted at a threshold of energy availability in regularly menstruating women. *The*

Journal of Clinical Endocrinology & Metabolism,
88(1), 297–311. https://doi.org/10.1210/jc.2002-020369

Loucks, A. B., Verdun, M., & Heath, E. M. (1998). Low energy availability, not stress of exercise, alters LH pulsatility in exercising women. *Journal of Applied Physiology,* *84*(1), 37–46. https://doi.org/10.1152/jappl.1998.84.1.37

Madell, R., & Nall, R. (2018, November 13). *Good fats vs. bad fats.* Healthline. https://www.healthline.com/health/heart-disease/good-fats-vs-bad-fats#bottom-line

Makni, M., Fetoui, H., Gargouri, N. K., Garoui, E. M., & Zeghal, N. (2011). Antidiabetic effect of flax and pumpkin seed mixture powder: Effect on hyperlipidemia and antioxidant status in alloxan diabetic rats. *Journal of Diabetes and Its Complications,* *25*(5), 339–345. https://doi.org/10.1016/j.jdiacomp.2010.09.001

Mancinelli, K. (n.d.). *15 tips to success on your intermittent fast.* Kristen Mancinelli MS, RD. http://kristenmancinelli.com/15-tips-succeed-on-intermittent-fast

Mann, D. (2013, April 30). *Is lack of sleep causing you to gain weight?* WebMD. https://www.webmd.com/sleep-disorders/features/lack-of-sleep-weight-gain

Martin, B., Mattson, M. P., & Maudsley, S. (2006). Caloric restriction and intermittent fasting: Two potential diets for successful brain aging. *Ageing Research*

Reviews, 5(3), 332–353.
https://doi.org/10.1016/j.arr.2006.04.002

Mayo Clinic Staff. (2020, December 8). *Counting calories: Get back to weight-loss basics.* Mayo Clinic. https://www.mayoclinic.org/healthy-lifestyle/weight-loss/in-depth/calories/art-20048065

McFarlane, S. I. (2009). Antidiabetic medications and weight gain: Implications for the practicing physician. *Current Diabetes Reports,* 9(3), 249–254. https://doi.org/10.1007/s11892-009-0040-7

Meyer, H. (2018, February). *Cauliflower English muffins.* EatingWell. https://www.eatingwell.com/recipe/262577/cauliflower-english-muffins/

Murtagh, E. M., Murphy, M. H., & Boone-Heinonen, J. (2010). Walking: the first steps in cardiovascular disease prevention. *Current Opinion in Cardiology,* 22(5), 490–496. https://doi.org/10.1097/hco.0b013e32833ce972

Napoli, N. (2018, March 1). *Regular walking may protect against heart failure post menopause.* American College of Cardiology. https://www.acc.org/about-acc/press-releases/2018/02/27/11/53/regular-walking-may-protect-against-heart-failure-post-menopause

The Nutrition Source. (2012, September 18). *Fats and cholesterol.* https://www.hsph.harvard.edu/nutritionsource/what-should-you-eat/fats-and-cholesterol/

O'Gallagher, G. (2016, July 12). *Intermittent fasting for teens - Is it safe?* Kinobody Fitness Systems. https://blog.kinobody.com/best-of/diet-nutrition-and-fasting/intermittent-fasting-for-teenagers/

Overweight calculator. (2019). Calculator.net. https://www.calculator.net/overweight-calculator.html

Patten, S. B., Williams, J. V. A., Lavorato, D. H., Khaled, S., & Bulloch, A. G. M. (2011). Weight gain in relation to major depression and antidepressant medication use. *Journal of Affective Disorders, 134*(1-3), 288–293. https://doi.org/10.1016/j.jad.2011.06.027

Petre, A. (2019, June 20). *"Calories in, calories out" — Does it really matter?* Healthline. https://www.healthline.com/nutrition/calories-in-calories-out

Santos, H. O., & Macedo, R. C. O. (2018). Impact of intermittent fasting on the lipid profile: Assessment associated with diet and weight loss. *Clinical Nutrition ESPEN, 24,* 14–21. https://doi.org/10.1016/j.clnesp.2018.01.002

Shai, I., Schwarzfuchs, D., Henkin, Y., Shahar, D. R., Witkow, S., Greenberg, I., Golan, R., Fraser, D., Bolotin, A., Vardi, H., Tangi-Rozental, O., Zuk-Ramot, R., Sarusi, B., Brickner, D., Schwartz, Z., Sheiner, E., Marko, R., Katorza, E., Thiery, J., & Fiedler, G. M. (2008). Weight loss with a low-carbohydrate, Mediterranean, or low-fat diet. *The New England Journal of Medicine, 359*(3), 229–241. https://doi.org/10.1056/NEJMoa0708681

Shin, B. K., Kang, S., Kim, D. S., & Park, S. (2018). Intermittent fasting protects against the deterioration of cognitive function, energy metabolism and dyslipidemia in Alzheimer's disease-induced estrogen deficient rats. *Experimental Biology and Medicine*, *243*(4), 334–343. https://doi.org/10.1177/1535370217751610

Spritzler, F. (2020, October 5). *Fat grams: How much fat should you eat per day?* Healthline. https://www.healthline.com/nutrition/how-much-fat-to-eat

Steinhilber, B. (2018, May 4). *Why walking is the most underrated form of exercise.* NBC News. https://www.nbcnews.com/better/health/why-walking-most-underrated-form-exercise-ncna797271

van Proeyen, K., Szlufcik, K., Nielens, H., Ramaekers, M., & Hespel, P. (2011). Beneficial metabolic adaptations due to endurance exercise training in the fasted state. *Journal of Applied Physiology (Bethesda, Md. : 1985)*, *110*(1), 236–245. https://doi.org/10.1152/japplphysiol.00907.2010

Vanderwall, C. (n.d.). *What is one reason that a high-carb diet makes me overeat and gain weight? Carbohydrates and weight loss.* Sharecare.https://www.sharecare.com/health/carbohydrates-weight-loss/high-carb-gain-weight

Waehner, P. (2020, January 21). *4 effective ways to track your weight loss progress.* Verywell Fit. https://www.verywellfit.com/ways-to-track-weight-loss-progress-1231581

Wang, Y., & Xu, D. (2017). Effects of aerobic exercise on lipids and lipoproteins. *Lipids in Health and Disease, 16*(1). https://doi.org/10.1186/s12944-017-0515-5

Wilkinson, M. J., Manoogian, E. N. C., Zadourian, A., Lo, H., Fakhouri, S., Shoghi, A., Wang, X., Fleischer, J. G., Navlakha, S., Panda, S., & Taub, P. R. (2020). Ten-hour time-restricted eating reduces weight, blood pressure, and atherogenic lipids in patients with metabolic syndrome. *Cell Metabolism, 31*(1), 92-104.e5. https://doi.org/10.1016/j.cmet.2019.11.004

Wnuk, A. (2018, July 13). *How does fasting affect the brain?* www.brainfacts.org. https://www.brainfacts.org/thinking-sensing-and-behaving/diet-and-lifestyle/2018/how-does-fasting-affect-the-brain-071318

Yetman, D. (2020, August 10). *Hydrostatic weighing: What it measures, how it works, when it's done.* Healthline. https://www.healthline.com/health/hydrostatic-weighing#how-its-done